Praise for *Gifts of the Heart...*

"The gifted surgeon shows us the power of purpose in the operating room, in life, and on the battlefield. Get ready to passionately pursue your purpose!"

—Greg Salciccioli, author of *The Enemies of Excellence*

"A spellbinding story that transports the reader from the orderly heart surgery operating room in Minnesota to the chaos of a battlefield outpost in Afghanistan as Dr. Kareem Afram struggles to learn and incorporate the lifesaving values of humility, gratitude, love, and persistence."

—Edward A. Lefrak, MD, author of *Cardiac Valve Prostheses* and Founder of Cardiac, Vascular, and Thoracic Surgery Associates

"Seeing the Operating Room, its players, and its patients dramatized in such a realistic and exciting fashion reaffirms the author's noble work."

—Patricia C Seifert, RN, author of *Cardiac Surgery*

"Hassan Tetteh's descriptions of battlefield operating theaters make M.A.S.H. look like a Sunday school picnic. And yet it is a moving portrait of pain, courage, and spiritual discovery that turns it into a coming-of-age story. A real page-turner."

—Richard H. Robbins, Ph.D., author of *Global Problems and the Culture of Capitalism*

"This extraordinary novel displays the dedication, sensitivity, and compassion that we all expect from our physicians—in this case, in the worst possible conditions, wartime Afghanistan.... Read it to be inspired!"

—Douglas R. Skopp, Ph.D., SUNY Distinguished Teaching Professor of History, *emeritus,* and author of *Shadows Walking: A Novel*

"*Gifts of the Heart* is a captivating read from start to finish. This book transports readers from the relatively safe harbors of daily life to harrowing moments that demand more than skill and expertise—they require 'Gifts of the Heart'—the ability to transcend self to live a life of service and love. Dr. Tetteh brings readers to the precipice of life that requires more than our skills and knowledge. The precipice requires our love and service. *Gifts of the Heart* leaves readers with a question: what decisions will we make that determine the life we live and lead?"

—Adelaide Schaeffer, President and CEO, Champions for Kids

Continued

"A powerful testimony to a profession that is life encompassing but incredibly rewarding for the devoted practitioner who performs intricate skilled procedures both from perspective of the critical need of the patient, but also a love of the work. It is clear the author captures emotional and moving experience to keep the reader spellbound. Real life experiences from both the operating theater and the battlefield highlight the fragility of life in both. A wonderful first novel.... I expect to see more of the same in the future."
  —Ceeya Patton Bolman, Program Director, Team Heart, Inc.

"Hassan Tetteh's first novel about the education—both in medicine and in life—of Dr. Kareem Afram reminds us that we must apply lessons of the heart in all we do. It's a required read for anyone who wants to make an impact on the world."
  —Mary Somers, MS, Associate Director of Admissions,
  Johns Hopkins Carey Business School

"A heartwarming and inspirational story of a combat surgeon healing and being healed through medicine and faith in the greater glory of God."
  —Rev. Christopher S. Fronk, Former 2D Marine Division (FWD) Chaplain

"This is a compelling journey into harm's way by a soldier and surgeon. Dr. Tetteh has taken that journey, and his story is an important one to hear and understand. The medical perspective on war deepens our appreciation for the difficult decisions and sacrifices our soldiers, their families, and the communities that have supported them have had to make and will continue to make as they heal."
  —David Sklar, MD, Distinguished Professor and Associate Dean Emeritus,
  University of New Mexico, author, *La Clinica: A Doctor's Journey Across Borders*

"The terrible casualties of the Iraq and Afghanistan wars have required courage, creativity, and endurance from the medical profession. This book tells the story from the perspective of a combat surgeon, facing life-or-death decisions in the operating room."
  —Linda J. Bilmes, Professor, Harvard Kennedy School, Co-author, *The Three Trillion Dollar War: The True Cost of the Iraq Conflict*

"This beautifully written story is a precious gift from the author's own heart on how each of us can live a more purposeful, more connected, life. Dr. Tetteh deftly blends immigrant upbringing, surgical achievement, military service, and restorative faith in God into a gripping spiritual allegory."
  —Charles Perry, MD, MBA, Managing Director at Dialectic Partners

Gifts

of the

Heart

A Novel

HASSAN A. TETTEH
with Foreword by
Christopher B. Dewing

Published in the United States by Tetteh Consulting Group (TCG Publishing), Bethesda, Maryland

This is a work of fiction. Names, characters, places, and incidents either are the product of the author's imagination or are used fictitiously. Any resemblance to actual persons, living or dead, events, or locales is entirely coincidental.

The views expressed in this article are those of the author and do not necessarily reflect the official policy or position of the U.S. Department of the Navy, U.S. Department of Defense, or the United States Government.

Scripture quotations are taken from:
The Holy Bible, New Living Translation, copyright 1996. Used by permission of Tyndale House Publishers, Inc., Wheaton, Illinois 60189. All rights reserved.

THE HOLY BIBLE: NEW INTERNATIONAL VERSION®. NIV®. Copyright © 1973, 1978, 1984 by Biblica. All rights reserved worldwide.

Library of Congress Cataloging-in-Publication Data
1. Physicians-Fiction 2. Fathers and Sons-Fiction 3. Brooklyn (New York, N.Y.)-Fiction 4. Sierra Leone-Fiction 5. Ghana-Fiction 6. Afghanistan-Fiction 7. Surgery-Fiction
ISBN: 978-0-578-12234-2

Cover Design by Steven Dana
Steven Dana is a nationally recognized book designer and can be contacted at www.stevendanapaintings.com

Printed in the United States of America
13 14 15 16 17—7 6 5 4 3 2 1

for Edmund Metzger Tetteh

Contents

◇

Foreword

IN THE FALL OF 2011, HASSAN AND I LIVED AND worked side-by-side in an austere United States Navy, Role 2, Forward Resuscitative Surgical Suite in Afghanistan. Our time there transformed us, both as surgeons and as men, and forged a lasting friendship and exchange of ideas that helped to inspire this book, Hassan's first novel. This book is not an autobiography, but the protagonist shares many of Hassan's fine qualities. Both men have a deep gratitude for the freedom and opportunity of the American Dream, a nuanced understanding of their cultural heritage, a poetic eye, and a surgeon's steady hand.

Prior to our deployment, I was stationed in San Diego as a Navy orthopaedic surgeon, specializing in sports injuries. Hassan worked as a Navy cardiothoracic surgeon at Bethesda/Walter Reed. Hassan's soft-spoken, well-spoken, bespectacled presence was a welcome contrast to the bluster and fluster of our six weeks of "training" at Camp Lejeune. We joined a group of surgeons, nurses, and corpsmen setting up tents, trialing gas masks, and firing assault rifles in the stifling humidity of a Carolina summer. We were all wary of what we would face in Afghanistan over the next seven months, and we were all homesick after fresh farewells to our families.

It took over ten days and a combination of civilian and military aircraft to get to our assigned forward operating base

(FOB), in a particularly "kinetic" corner of the Helmand river valley of Southwest Afghanistan. We clambered out of the belly of our massive transport helicopter, struggling under the weight of our combat gear, onto the rocky airfield and dragged our bags towards the medical tents, just visible over the HESCO barriers. We were all cursing the blistering heat and dust and the fact that no one had come out to give us a hand with our gear, when we saw the Army DUSTOFF helicopters coming onto the base low and fast.

The existing Navy Surgical Team, that we had come to replace, cleared us to the side. Their corpsmen sprinted out to the Blackhawks and came back carrying a limp and mangled body. The Marine's legs were gone, and what was left of his thighs was beyond recognition, a tangle of ripped, burned, bloody muscle and bone. We stood there, frozen for that split second, by shock, horror, and fear. Then, abruptly, the Marine sat bolt upright and glared at us, before collapsing into unconsciousness as he was rushed into the tent. Hassan and I struggled out of our flak jackets and Kevlar helmets and pushed inside.

I will never forget our "operating room," an old, sagging GP tent with just enough space to accommodate one litter stand, an anesthesia machine, and basic surgical equipment. No matter how much we cleaned it, dust found its way into and onto everything. With all the lights on, it still felt dark, and the temperature rarely dipped below one hundred degrees. Our patients came to us straight from the battlefield, in severe shock from the massive blood loss of multiple amputations.

Foreword

We operated, two surgeons on each side of the table, in a race to definitively control bleeding. The anesthesia team used rapid infusers to replace volume, often using fresh, whole blood from a "Walking Blood Bank" of Marines and Soldiers, eager to help us by donating their own blood on the spot.

The urgency and austerity of the surgery was a shock to all of us, but especially to Hassan, whose cardiothoracic training and practice emphasized elegance, precision, and technical perfection. After a few cases, we had all accepted the brutality and frugality of battlefield surgery. We had no choice; lives were hanging on the balance. We focused on cheating death. We counted on each other and clung to our Faith. We never lost a patient in the tent. If they came in with a pulse, they left stable and strong enough to begin the many stages of their MEDEVAC homeward.

Some patients died just before the courageous Army DUSTOFF crews could get them to us, and we tried everything we could to bring them back. Hassan opened their chests, guiding us through cardiac massage and advanced resuscitation. But their wounds and blood loss were nonsurvivable. Our "Hero" patients were meticulously prepared and their bodies were draped with our Ensign. We all lined the honor guard procession from the tent to the flight line, standing at attention until the helicopters lifted away to the south.

In between cases, we fought off the anxiety and anticipation of the next trauma arrival with exercise, conversation, reading, and prayer. Access to the Internet was limited, so Hassan and I leased a small satellite system from a British vendor at the closest big base, and spent the better part of a week crawling around on top of the Quad containers behind our medical tents, running cable, tracking satellites, and tuning our dish. Our WiFi was a huge morale booster for the whole medical team.

When Hassan was selected to leave early, we all felt a great loss. I knew him well enough by then to empathize with his quiet quest to integrate the varied challenges of his deployment to the Helmand. On the day before he left, Hassan shed some dusty tears as we shared memories of our patients and considered the magnitude of their sacrifices. We prayed that they would find the courage and determination to heal from their wounds.

We have since returned to our busy surgical practices in the Navy. We have both seen our patients on campus, and many more like them, bravely learning to walk again, this time on state-of-the-art prosthetic limbs. We are grateful to know that our early hours with these Warriors in our small tent gave life to their remarkable and inspirational work of recovery.

Nunc Coepi
Now we begin...

Christopher B. Dewing, MD
San Diego, California

PART I

To Heal

◇

Urgency

NOTHING COMPARES TO THE THRILL OF SAVING a life. Pilots may have their flying machines and g-forces, astronauts their space, and even race car drivers their NASCAR, but surgeons experience the intangible feeling of making a difference between life and death—and, in the balance, save lives.

For Dr. Kareem Afram, one especially memorable life-saving moment occurred in the final years of his cardiothoracic fellowship, the period when a surgeon's skills are polished and refined, his instinct sharpened, and his hubris at its apogee.

From humble Brooklyn beginnings, Dr. Afram had completed college in three years, graduated from medical school at the top of his class, and trained as a general surgeon before traveling the Pacific Ocean as a U.S. Navy medical officer. Afram had joined the Navy reserves after 9/11, feeling the patriotic volunteerism that embraced many in America after that tragedy.

After joining the Navy, Kareem Afram decided he wanted to be more than "just a surgeon"; he wanted to be a *heart* surgeon. He had mastered all operations of the abdomen, and as a chief resident had completed one of surgery's technically most difficult operation—the Whipple procedure—more times than any other trainee in the history of his hospital's training program. His grace in the operating room earned him the nickname "Dr. Elegant." He once told a fellow surgeon, "I want my hands to do great things. In the chest is where I want to be—in that cage that seems so forbidden."

All doctors experience failure and face the unexpected moment when good judgment and action make all the difference between life and death. Dr. Afram faced those moments and overcame failure many times. He was a seasoned crisis manager and consummate physician. Any patient would be fortunate to have him as their doctor.

Near the end of his cardiothoracic fellowship, which took place in Minnesota, one of his patients was a Mr. Pine, a large man who had difficulty all his life finding shirts to fit. His large head sat on his shoulders without regard for the neck. His personality was just as large as his robust body—he was fun, the kind of person you'd want as your wingman on a night out on the town.

Pine had become Dr. Afram's patient because of an aortic aneurysm, a ballooning of the largest vessel that carries blood from the heart to the rest of the body; his heart also had a diseased aortic valve. His aorta was on the fatal verge of rupture when Dr. Afram operated on him. Afram replaced Pine's diseased aorta with a composite graft of Dacron polyester fabric and inserted a new heart valve.

After surgery, Dr. Afram declared that Mr. Pine would be "good for another hundred thousand miles." The procedure was a success. Pine spent a day in ICU and soon was recovering in the surgical wards, awaiting discharge.

During morning rounds on his third day after surgery, Pine's nurse frantically called out into the hallway, "Help, we need help in here! Mr. Pine can't breathe!"

Indeed, when Afram arrived to his patient's room, the once jovial Mr. Pine was in trouble. He muttered, "I, I ca—I, I can't brea—" His heart rate and blood pressure were elevated, and he was pale and ashen.

"We need help in here, now—get the crash cart!" Dr. Afram quickly realized, as other providers came rushing to the bedside, that Pine was having cardiac tamponade, a life-threatening condition in which the heart fails because of outside compression from blood and fluid.

Dr. Afram did the clinical calculus. In Pine's case, his problem was caused by slow postoperative bleeding; now all that blood had nowhere to go in his chest and was pressing on the heart, restricting its motion. "We need to get to the operating room now," Afram ordered. "Call the charge nurse and clear a path to the OR!"

Suddenly Pine's eyes rolled to the back of his head and he became unresponsive.

"No pulse, no blood pressure, no signs of life!" a nurse screamed. At that moment, all eyes were on Afram. "Open the crash cart!" he said. "Sterile gloves, gown, and cut-down tray!" This tray contained all the items Afram needed to perform surgery at the bedside, including wire cutters to open up Pine's chest.

Conditions were less than ideal, with poor lighting and the struggle against confusion and panic. Still there was superfluity of movement and personnel. Afram made requests, the team assigned tasks, and everyone focused on some part of Pine's now limp body. Afram focused on the chest. It had to be opened, and the blood had to be evacuated from around his heart if he were to have any chance for survival. It had to be done *now*.

With scalpel in hand, Afram sliced through the incision. He parted Pine's now healing wound and cut the wires that were placed just days ago to hold his chest together. Blood erupted from the new opening.

Every surgeon dreads this moment—operating under poor light, in an emergency, and under duress. Excellent surgeons live for this moment—a chance to use all that has been learned over years of training and long hours of arduous work, bringing it all together when it matters most. Dr. Afram was a pro, and he performed with equanimity.

With wires cut, Pine's sternum was pulled apart. More blood poured from his chest and oozed down his sides onto the sheets. "Retractor!" Afram placed this device to keep the chest open and expose the heart that was hiding in its forbidden cage. For the uninitiated, and even for the seasoned, the scene was amazing. Anxious gazes and stares were fixed on Afram and the open chest of the lifeless Mr. Pine.

Pine's heart was now in plain view, a sleeping organ enveloped by clotted blood. Afram reached in. "Suction!"

He scooped out the clotted blood that had trapped the indispensable pump, but the maneuver was not enough. There was no activity. No circulation. No life.

Dr. Afram delicately held the heart in both his hands and squeezed. His cardiac massage began to move the life-giving blood around Pine's body. "We're in," confirmed the anesthesiologist, after slipping in a breathing tube to support the airway. By this time, a team was breathing for him, and providers were administering drugs and fluid—all in an effort to revive this man. But the heart was still quiet.

Afram then remembered a bold move that had worked in a similar case. "One amp of Epi," he called out. He injected the full syringe of adrenaline directly into Pine's heart.

Nothing—no activity, no movement, no life.

Afram massaged the heart again, simulating what the heart would do on its own if it could. He could feel the thrill of blood flowing from one chamber to the next as he squeezed the limp pump. Then, under his hands, Afram felt a little wiggle, a coordinated collective movement of the heart's muscle cells and some activity.

"He's fibrillating!" Afram announced. The heart's motions were unsynchronized, but there *was* movement—and now there was hope!

"Paddles," ordered Afram. He placed the large spoon-shaped paddles around the heart. "Charge...I'm clear, you're clear...Shock!"

Pine's entire body moved with the discharge of the current.

"No response, still fibrillating," Afram declared. The massaging continued. "Charge," he repeated. "I'm clear, you're clear…Shock!" Then a third time, and then a fourth.

And then…success. Pine's heart was back. He had a rhythm and a pulse.

With Afram's hand still in Pine's open chest, the team cleared a path through the crowded hospital hallways to the elevators. With Afram alongside, Pine was rushed into the operating room. There the bleeding would be brought under control and his condition stabilized.

Within hours, Pine's chest was closed again, and he was on his way back to the Intensive Care Unit. That evening he was moving around and breathing on his own again.

The next morning he was up and out of bed and asked Afram, "Doc, what happened?"

Overflowing with accomplishment, Dr. Afram responded, "Mr. Pine, you're a lucky man. You had a little leak, but you're fixed now and still good for many more miles. There must be a reason you're still alive!"

This man soon went home, and Dr. Afram often wondered if Mr. Pine—and patients like him, who narrowly avoid death—ever discover the reason for their extended gift of life.

Reflecting on his own life's path, Afram held many hearts in his hand and imagined the purpose of the life that was supported by the perfect pump. Dr. Afram was sure of his purpose. Years before, standing before a group of medical students, he had announced, "I always knew I wanted to be a heart surgeon. I wanted to operate on the beating heart and do what many said I could never do. I wanted the challenge, and now I've achieved what seemed impossible just a short while ago. As a surgeon, I want to steady the shake and line the needle straight, and I plan to be the best."

It took many years for Dr. Afram to develop his affirmation. And like Mr. Pine, Afram had to come close to death and be rescued by grace before he realized his own true calling.

◇

Freetown

"UNLESS YOU KNOW THE ROAD YOU'VE COME from," an African proverb says, "you cannot know where you are going."

If Kareem Afram had been born in his mother's hometown village of southwest Freetown, Sierra Leone, he would have known of beautiful beaches that welcomed returning African slaves from America. He would have played on hillsides overlooking the Atlantic, and he would have spoken Creole. Kareem would have learned more about his mother's family and her eight siblings who left her behind in Africa to move to Beirut, Lebanon with their father's family. Kareem's mother, Miriam, was separated from her older siblings because she was the last of her father's children. Miriam never knew him, because he died before she was born. Chance and timing ensured that her life would be much different from that of her brothers and sisters.

Miriam spent much of her life trying to learn about her mysterious Lebanese father, and ultimately would name her last-born child, Kareem, after the father she never knew.

Her mother, Dayo, was a beautiful Krio woman of Yoruba descent. When Lebanese businessmen arrived in Sierra Leone for trade in the country's great diamond resources, they were invariably attracted to the Krio women. Dayo's name means "joy," yet the early death of her father snatched fortune and happiness from her and her mother.

Miriam was fair-skinned, with long straight hair; her appearance was the equal product of her African mother and Lebanese father. She treasured the one picture she had of her mother, Dayo, that captured the black woman wearing a white dress and headpiece. Her mother's eyes were seductively haunting, set in a smileless face lined with age and loss from years without a husband and her children.

But instead of being born in his mother's village, Kareem would live a different kind of life because of a courageous journey his mother took across the Atlantic in 1954. Over a decade after Miriam's journey, Kareem would be born in Brooklyn and grow up playing in the streets that lined this city overlooking the other side of the Atlantic. Indeed, Dr. Kareem Afram would travel down a different path because of the road his mother Miriam took.

Cultivation

MIRIAM ZAYD ARRIVED TO THE UNITED STATES in the mid-1950s with her best friend, Hadiya Queen. The two girls left Sierra Leone with plans to travel to the United Kingdom, but were persuaded by an aggressive ticket agent and a lower fare at the last minute to change ships for one heading to the Unites States. They were among the last immigrants to land at Ellis Island.

Miriam left Sierra Leone—or "Salone," as it was called—searching for something bigger than she had known there. Although she was only sixteen and Hadiya just two years older when they settled in New York, they both passed for much older women.

Their early years in Brooklyn were wild. They went from rent house to rent house, often dodging landlords seeking unpaid rent. They held odd jobs from cleaning to serving tables, and anything else that would pay.

There was a growing African immigrant population in Brooklyn, and they found a community of friends among other young Africans who had left familiar homes in West Africa for the promise of America. Miriam had her mother's beauty without the lines of pain and loss. She was called "Mimi," a free spirit. She smoked cigarettes with Hadiya, and they complemented each other in every way. They were in constant search of adventure and a new beginning. America was the land of opportunity, they were told; they both learned it was a place where anything was possible.

Eventually Miriam landed steady employment as a housekeeper for a wealthy, well-educated Manhattan businessman and his family. Miriam was enamored of her employer's wealth and what she saw in the rich upper-east-side neighborhood where she worked. Never formally educated, her experience on the streets of New York provided her with an education in survival. She began to save her money, and she realized from her exposure to a world of wealth that there was money to be made in America.

Her long straight hair inherited from her Lebanese father always required extra care, and she had long ago developed a special skill of styling and braiding it, and doing it also for other women's hair back in Freetown. In America she learned that women would pay her well for this talent that she had developed out of necessity. She became an especially shrewd businesswoman, making extra income by styling and cutting hair in her apartment.

Her friend Hadiya found work as a model and started to travel away from New York for long weekends, then eventually spent months away in Europe and Canada. She soon married a French exporter she met in Canada, and settled in Quebec. Miriam and her friend always remained close and spoke whenever they could.

New York's African immigrant community continued to grow explosively in the 1970s. Miriam's reputation as a hair stylist also kept growing, and she became quite popular among Africans in Brooklyn.

Ten years after her arrival in New York, Miriam was still young and even more beautiful. She was now a woman of the city, and she had become an American citizen. This made her even more attractive to African men seeking a permanent stay in the United States. Miriam never looked back to "Salone" and Freetown; her love affair with America only grew stronger as the years passed.

Her romance with America was abruptly shaken by news of her mother's death back in Sierra Leone, deeply affecting Miriam. She had not gone back to Freetown for all those years. All she possessed of her beloved Dayo was a black-and-white photo, and her only trip home in over ten years would be to bury her mother. Miriam's guilt was overwhelming. Throughout her decade in America, she'd thought only of advancing herself, yet she felt she'd actually achieved very little in all those years. And now she had no mother as well as no father. Her friend Hadiya was married and had her own family, with children of her own. But Miriam's remaining family—her brothers and sisters—were lost to her in Lebanon.

She was very alone in America, a world that was now so very different.

Then a mutual friend in New York introduced her to Kwame Afram, a man named after Kwame Nkrumah, the visionary leader and first president of Ghana who worked so hard for unity among African nations. Kwame Afram was a dreamer. He'd come to America with little skill, seeking riches and fame. He determined to make his mark in the world. A tall, spirited, handsome man from Cape Coast, Ghana, he'd arrived in America only a year before meeting Miriam and avoided all traditional routes of employment because he was not a U.S. citizen. Not having citizenship was a great liability at the time, with serious potential for arrest and deportation.

Miriam's romance with Kwame was not storybook. She was lonely and recovering from loss, while he was a charming companion who saw an opportunity in her vulnerability and an easy path to citizenship. They were married in New York's City Hall seven months after meeting.

Miriam's first and second pregnancies ended in miscarriages. Years of fast city life and smoking had taken their toll both physically and now emotionally. Miriam and Kwame's indifference and frosty relationship grew even chillier with the failed attempts to conceive, and the reality of their unfulfilled dreams haunted them both.

Miriam kept working as a housekeeper and styled hair in the evenings and weekends. Kwame had random factory jobs and eventually began driving a taxi once he obtained his license. His great plans for fame and riches were dashed away in the long hours driving through the city. Except for fleeting moments in the night, Miriam and Kwame saw very little of each other.

In 1971, a year before John Lennon released his political album *Some Time in New York City*, Miriam and Kwame's son

Kareem Afram was born. Miriam's void was immediately filled with her new son. She named him Kareem in tribute to her lost father, much to the chagrin of Kwame. With his Catholic background, Kwame worried about having a Catholic son named Kareem, but Miriam wouldn't yield.

The Catholic Church was strongly influential in Kwame's hometown of Cape Coast back in Ghana. The roots of this influence went back to the Portuguese explorers and settlers who brought the Catholic faith to West Africa five centuries earlier. More recently, the church's Second Vatican Council of 1962–1965 had caused a groundswell of Catholic growth in the region. Catholic churches peppered the hills overlooking the Atlantic. This faith had been passed from generation to generation down to Kwame's family. Both his parents were Catholic, and he had attended Catholic elementary and secondary school.

Now with his own son in New York, Kwame pledged to Miriam that Kareem would go to Catholic school just as he had.

In America, Kwame embraced the music of the Beatles, Motown, Bob Marley, and others because he identified with their lyrics and political messages of the day. Music eased his frustrations with episodic unemployment. He believed in the music that spoke out against social injustice and the discrimination which he was sure prevented him from being successful.

Although somewhat supportive of his wife's work, Kwame quietly resented Miriam's entrepreneurial success and her ease with finding employment, and he was increasingly concerned that their son would face similar challenges as he grew up. He determined, however, to shield his son as much as possible from the real world. As Kareem grew up, Kwame determined to offer him continual encouragement, as he reflected on the fact of having a son who was "made in the USA."

Kareem unquestionably brought both Miriam and Kwame closer to each other, at least initially. Miriam was happy, and an unfamiliar type of joy was now part of her life. For both of them, the personal dreams that once seemed vanquished now felt possible again. For Miriam especially, but also to some degree for Kwame, their American dream could now be realized through their son, Kareem.

Miriam sang lullabies to Kareem, and whispered to him, "This land is a rich land. In this country, oh, anything is possible!" She held her son tightly, as she looked tenderly into his eyes and dreamed. Miriam couldn't remember or imagine what she did before Kareem came into her life. She gave up much of her old life and even stopped smoking. All of her energy was focused on her son.

Kwame played the music of the day for his son. He loved the song "Angela" and the militant picture of Angela Davis on the cover of Lennon's *Some Time in New York City*. Kwame would sing the chorus: "They gave you sunshine...They gave you everything but the jailhouse key...They gave you everything but equality."

To Heal

Angela Davis was a worldwide phenomenon and hero to many in Africa, and especially in Ghana. Kwame hoped that as a social consciousness developed in America, things would be better for his son, Kareem. His American-born son would not be an outsider and immigrant like his parents. Miriam and Kwame had come to America with nothing more than hope and dreams. Their dreams were to make a better life for themselves, and for years that hope seemed to fade away along with any possibility of ever achieving their goals. Kareem restored hope for both of them, and he gave them a renewed faith in dreams—and to some extent, in America.

◇

Red Shoes

"WHO'S THE DOCTOR WITH THOSE RED SHOES?" the nurse asked.

It's the question many would ask when they first encountered Dr. Afram, whose red clogs were his trademark.

He first wore them in trauma service during his surgical residency in New York City, choosing the color because blood was always falling on his shoes. His combination ensemble of royal blue scrubs, red clogs, and long cape-like white coat made him look like a superhero, and he loved the look. He felt invincible in the outfit, so he stuck with it. Afram's red clogs and confidence carried him through hundreds of cases—thousands of hours of patient care, rounds, and operations.

On one auspicious day in the hospital, Afram heard overhead the dreaded announcement, "Code Blue...sixth floor, room 612—*Code Blue!*"

That was the cardiac floor, Afram knew, where all his patients were. He glanced at his patient census list and exhaled a sigh of relief; he didn't have a patient in that room. *But some poor person is leaving this world*, he thought. That was the reality of surgery. It was "okay" to have bad things happen to patients as long as they weren't *your* patients. Bad things happening to a surgeon's own personal patients were never okay.

Still, Afram's instincts were to trust but always verify, and he headed up to the room on the sixth floor just to make sure. On arrival, there was pandemonium. A crowd of nurses, doctors, and bystanders were in the room around the bedside of a patient who was clearly in trouble and dying. The patient was as blue as Afram's scrubs. Two doctors were at the patient's head, trying to ventilate him. They forced air into his mouth with an air bag and mask, while trying to place a plastic endotracheal breathing tube in the patient's airway so he could get much-needed oxygen to reverse his color and save him from death.

From the patient's doorway, Afram assessed the situation quickly. Multiple attempts were already being made to place the plastic endotracheal tube in the patient's throat, and with each successive attempt, the patient's airway was traumatized further. It made each additional attempt to place the tube almost impossible with the increased swelling and traumatic bleeding. The scene was desperate, and the patient was slipping away.

"We need a cut-down tray, now!" Afram asserted forcefully, with confident arrogance in his voice. He knew exactly what needed to be done and went to work. He knew the only way the patient could now survive was to cut through his neck and place a breathing tube directly through the windpipe.

"Keep ventilating," he told the doctors at the head of the bed. "Let's get a shoulder roll—we need some extra light in here." He skillfully felt for the familiar landmarks on the neck and found the spot to cut.

"Betadine, get an airway tube ready," Afram ordered as he donned surgical gloves. With a calm and steady hand, he reached for the scalpel in the tray and made a deliberate vertical cut through the skin, deep enough to scratch the windpipe. He wiped the blood from the skin to clear his view. Afram then advanced his finger through the wound to hold his spot—his finger was in between two tracheal rings.

"I feel the tracheal rings," he confirmed. "Keep ventilating."

He reached for the scalpel again, then made another stab at the windpipe, cutting in between the cartilaginous rings of the trachea. In one motion of his hand, Afram spun the scalpel around his index finger and thumb and advanced the blunt back of the scalpel through the trachea to expand the hole for the breathing tube. A gush of air and blood erupted from the hole in the patient's neck, as the doctors continued to bag the patient through the mask.

"Quick," Afram called, "I need the tube—hand me the breathing tube." He grabbed the plastic endotracheal tube and advanced it through the fresh hole. He hooked up the new airway to oxygen, and the patient immediately regained his pink color.

Afram secured the tube and called out, "Get the operating room ready!" The patient was now stable. As Afram made his way to the door and passed a witness, he heard an inquisitive whisper: "Who was that doctor in the red shoes?" Afram's red clogs struck again, and a great save was made.

He walked down the hall beaming from the adrenaline rush. He smiled, thinking, *Superman!*

◇

Dad's Lesson

HAVING TO WAIT IN THE DOCTOR'S OFFICE WAS Kareem's least favorite activity as a child. Finally seeing the doctor, however, was a treat.

Kareem's earliest memory of his family physician, Dr. Lloyd, involved waiting in a large room for hours, then waiting some more in the smaller room before finally seeing the doctor.

"How are you?" the doctor would say. "You're growing so big!" Dr. Lloyd was tall and confident, a West Indian man full of life with a thick accent and a knack for making patients laugh and feel good. He wore large brown-framed glasses, and a thick curly mustache outlined his smile. What impressed Kareem most was the doctor's long, white, crisp lab coat, with cursive script embossed on the chest that read: "Byron S. Lloyd, MD."

Dr. Lloyd practiced the same routine for years. He placed his hand on Kareem's shoulder and squeezed. He then asked, "You eating? You look too skinny, boy—skin and bones! How are Mummy and Dad?"

"Okay," Kareem answered.

"You doing okay in school—studying hard, eh?"

While the questions kept coming from Dr. Lloyd, he pulled out a tongue depressor from his white coat. "Say ahhh."

"Ahhh," Kareem complied, choking on the taste of stale wood.

"You cleaning your ears, boy?" the doctor asked as he looked inside them.

Then he listened to Kareem's chest with a stethoscope. "Kareem, take a deep breath in, and hold it," he instructed. "Breathe out again...deep breath and hold...breathe out." Hands and stethoscope skillfully glided back and forth across Kareem's chest as if the doctor were following a road map. Kareem flinched slightly each time the cold bell of the doctor's instrument touched his skin.

Dr. Lloyd always ended the routine by placing the stethoscope ear ports to Kareem's ears so he could listen to his own heartbeat. This was a treat, and the part Kareem loved most. Like the lollipop the nurse handed him upon leaving, Kareem always looked forward to hearing his own heartbeat.

"Why is my heart beating so hard?" Kareem would ask, feeling the pounding muscle against his chest. Kareem didn't realize it at the time, but his pounding heart muscle would be central to everything in his life.

"Why, you want it to beat soft?" Dr. Lloyd questioned.

"No!" answered Kareem.

Then Dr. Lloyd revealed his classic smile under his curly mustache and told Kareem, "Okay, boy, you all good, and I'll see you next year." Kareem and his mom would leave the office passing dozens of people in the waiting room.

Kareem once asked, "Are all these people waiting to see Dr. Lloyd?"

"Yes," she responded. "He's a very good doctor, and he helps people."

"How much money do doctors make?" Kareem asked.

"They get paid quite well," his mother answered.

"Wow!" Kareem whispered to himself. "What an easy job! All Dr. Lloyd ever does is ask me to say 'Ahhh,' listen to my heart, and then say I'm fine."

Kareem convinced himself at an early age that he wanted to be a doctor when he grew up, just like Dr. Lloyd. When he told this to his mother, Miriam did everything in her power to help him. Miriam had never graduated from high school, but she was street-smart, and through her employer she had witnessed what the power of education can do. She insisted that Kareem get a good education, and she fought for this at all times.

"Remember what I always told you, Kareem," she would say. "In this country, anything is possible. As long as you have an education and work hard, you can do anything you want in America."

The seeds of medicine were firmly planted in Kareem's young mind, and years of Catholic elementary school served to nurture him and provided him with a good foundation. The kind but firm nuns instilled faith and the fear of God in young Kareem. He questioned everything, and his teachers inspired a love of science and cultivated his curiosity. The priests taught young Kareem about the duty of service as an altar boy, and he learned about their important work of counseling those in need. Kareem attended Sunday Mass regularly and would often go by himself when his parents couldn't attend. Kareem's mother did all she could, working extra hours and styling hair with each spare hour to help pay for Kareem's education, and she encouraged him constantly.

Kareem's dad—like many in his hometown Cape Coast farming village—was heavily influenced by the church and was a great storyteller. Kwame used stories to teach Kareem lessons, as well as to scare him with punishment from God when Kareem misbehaved. Thanks to his own father, Kareem could recite many of Aesop's fables by the age of seven, and tell the moral behind each one.

"Kareem, I'll send you away to work on the farm if you misbehave," his father warned. He related stories of growing up in Cape Coast. He told young Kareem about his experience in school and the lessons he learned in the Bible. He described Africa vividly.

"I was third male child of nine children—*nine children,*" he said with pride. "We were a fishing family. My mom and dad wanted me to grow up and be a fisherman too, and to know how to survive on the sea.

"When I was nine years old, I went out on a fishing trip with my father. I thought we were just going out for a simple fishing trip, but the trip was actually a test! Not long after leaving the shore, I became violently ill. For hours I vomited and was seasick. I begged my father to go back to shore, but he wouldn't listen. We spent days on the sea. And I was a big disappointment to my father, because I didn't have what it took to be a fisherman."

There was sadness in Kwame's voice. "So my father sent me away to live with my auntie on her farm. This hurt me, but it was a blessing to be sent away, because in living on a farm, I learned a lot about life."

He opened his hands to show his rough palms to Kareem. "You see, when you work on a farm, you have to use your hands every day, and wake up early and work long hours all day. Your entire harvest depends on how much work you put in at the beginning. The work in the beginning is always the most important."

"Everyone on the farm, including me, worked to prepare the soil and plow the ground and then plant the seeds." He acted out these actions for Kareem. "Then we had to make sure we fertilized and watered the crops and pulled out the weeds."

Kwame concluded, "Yes, I learned a lot about life when I worked on the farm."

Kareem rolled his eyes in boredom. He was never interested in these stories about his father's farm life in faraway Africa, or in the questions his father asked about farms and life. Kareem's plan was to be a doctor, not a farmer. Besides, there were no farms in Brooklyn!

Kwame insisted that Kareem help out around the house, and he always gave Kareem tasks to do. Sometimes the young Kareem would respond, "I can't, Dad; it's too hard."

Then Kwame would tell his son, "Stop! Kareem, you need to remove this word *can't* from your vocabulary. On the farm, we would never say we can't feed the animals, or we can't plant the seeds, or we can't water the crops, or we can't pull the weeds. Because if we believed that, there would be no harvest, and we would have no food! There is no such word as *can't!*"

Even as Kwame lectured his son, he recognized his own hypocrisy. For he looked in the mirror each day, and reflecting back was the face of a man who couldn't fulfill his dreams of riches in America. Still, he longed for and prayed for his son to be a better man than he was. So he pressed his son constantly.

"You see," he told Kareem, "*can't* doesn't make the crops grow, and *can't* doesn't help you in life. There is no such word as *can't.*"

Kareem resented the lessons, stories, and advice his father offered. His dad was only a taxi cab driver, not a physician like Dr. Lloyd.

After years of Catholic elementary school, Kwame and Miriam could no longer afford to send Kareem to the more expensive Catholic middle school. Kareem experienced a very different education as he transitioned into a public middle school. He had been sheltered in Catholic school; now he was exposed to an entirely different system. The environment was no longer nurturing, he had few friends, and he kept to himself.

Soon after his arrival in the new school, Kareem was asked by a teacher, "What is it that you want to be when you grow up?"

Kareem, always encouraged by his mother and his Catholic school teachers, confidently responded, "I want to be a doctor."

The teacher seemed shocked by Kareem's answer. He crossed his hands, frowned, and raised his eyebrows. He squared his shoulders and looked at young Kareem, then said sarcastically, "You *really* want to be a doctor? You do know you need to finish middle school, and you have to finish high school, and not many kids in your neighborhood graduate from high school. Then you have to go to college for four years. Then you have to go to medical school for another four years. Then after all that, you have to do something called a residency."

Having described such an onerous path ahead for this precocious teenager, the teacher then asked, "Are you sure, Kareem, that's what you want to do when you grow up?"

Kareem remembered his experience in grade school, his mother's assertion about America, and his father's lessons about the word *can't*. "Yes," was his timid answer to his teacher.

Kareem wasn't entirely sure he would ever become a doctor after hearing this almost impossible course outlined by the teacher, but he remembered at that moment the two gifts his parents gave him. He knew what he wanted in his heart, and he remembered his faith.

Shortly after Kareem's sixteenth birthday, his father died from a heart attack. The doctors told Miriam and Kareem, "There was nothing we could do to save him. We are very sorry." He was only fifty-five years old.

Kareem couldn't find tears to cry on the day of his father's funeral. He was in shock. He questioned why the doctors couldn't do anything to save his father. *What kind of doctors were they? Doctors are supposed to be like Dr. Lloyd, and help people.*

Kareem had to face all at once the reality of no longer having a father, of suddenly being the man of the house, and of no longer having anyone talk to him about life on the farm. At every opportunity, Kareem worked hard to prove himself.

His departure from the structured Catholic school environment had exposed him to a whole new world. Initially keeping to himself, he soon embraced his new freedoms in his new school environment.

Kareem's mother, always a hard worker, was losing her influence on her teenage son as he came of age in inner-city Brooklyn, exposed to new friends. Although Kareem maintained focus on his academic work, he sought more social independence, which often placed him at odds with his mother. Miriam and Kareem argued often. She was struggling with the loss of her husband—the man she had grown to love and rely on—and the new reality of raising her independent son by herself.

To Heal

Without the presence of his father's spiritual influence and with the loss of religious structure, Kareem changed. He stopped his routine Mass attendance because he no longer saw the point. Kareem thought God had taken his father from him. After all his father's lessons about the farm, praying, and hard work, his father had died with nothing, as far as Kareem was concerned.

"I'm going to be something greater than my father," Kareem resolved. "I will be the kind of doctor who saves people that have heart attacks, even when God can't."

When three years had passed since his father's death, Kareem rediscovered a one-page letter written to him from his father. Kareem had received it from his dad at the time of his first retreat in Catholic school. That day was supposed to be a day of spiritual reflection, but all Kareem remembered of it was playing football with his friends.

Returning from the retreat, Kareem set the letter aside and had forgotten it ever since. Now, as he prepared to enter adulthood, he came across it again. The letter was very special, and even magical, because it reminded him of his father. Reading it, Kareem could almost hear his father's voice telling him another story:

Dear Kareem:

At this stage in your life you're beginning to realize that life is full of many beginnings and endings. Your mother and I are proud of you, and we want you to know that we are always with you. Although this note is short, you will find that if you read its references it is quite long indeed.

(On marriage:) Genesis 1:27–28— "So God created people in his own image; God patterned them after himself; male and female he created them. God blessed them and told them, 'Multiply and fill the earth and subdue it. Be masters over the fish and birds and all the animals.'"

(On children:) Psalm 127:3–5— "Children are a gift from the LORD; they are a reward from him. Children born to a young man are like sharp arrows in a warrior's hands. How happy is the man whose quiver is full of them!"

(On the duty of parents:) Deuteronomy 6:5–7— "You must love the LORD your God with all your heart, all your soul, and all your strength. And you must commit yourselves wholeheartedly to these commands I am giving you today. Repeat them again and again to your children."

(On a father's responsibility:) Ephesians 6:4— "And now a word to you fathers. Don't make your children angry by the way you treat them. Rather, bring them up with the discipline and instruction approved by the Lord."

(On life's challenges:) Luke 9:62— "No one who puts his hand to the plow and looks back is fit for service in the kingdom of God."

(On children's responsibility:) Deuteronomy 24:16— "Parents must not be put to death for the sins of their children, nor the children for the sins of their parents. Those worthy of death must be executed for their own crimes."

(On bad associations:) 1 Corinthians 15:33— "Don't be fooled by those who say such things, for 'bad company corrupts good character.'"

Love, Dad

Kareem read the letter over and over, and would treasure it throughout his life.

◇

Gift of Life

DR. KAREEM AFRAM WAS AT THE TOP OF HIS career when he met her.

Afram was now on the faculty at the best hospital in the Twin Cities of Minnesota, with a special practice in heart and lung transplantation and in treating advanced heart disease. Afram had moved to Minnesota for his heart surgery fellowship after his surgical training in New York, followed by a brief shipboard tour with the Navy. Afram was still a reserve officer and worked once a month with the reserve unit at the Minnesota Armory.

He always vividly remembered the day he met Hiral. He had been through three straight days of heart and lung transplants. In seventy-two hours Afram had traveled thousands of miles, as far north as Canada and as far south as Mississippi, harvesting organs for transplantation. He was delirious from fatigue, but he was instantly awakened when he saw Hiral for the first time.

She was a nutritionist at the hospital, in charge of all of the nutrition services for surgical patients. Recently hired from grad school in Minnesota, she had been born in Southern California but grew up in India. Hiral's friends teased her for moving from the warmest part of the country to coldest, and her parents rarely visited her from India. Hiral's father would complain, "*Mera bachcha*, my baby, *jaan,* Hiral…Minnesota is too cold!"

Hiral was adventurous, and she actually enjoyed the Minnesota winters. Immediately after graduation, her job as director of a major surgical service line gave her a great opportunity to make a real difference with patients.

The first time Afram's eyes met Hiral's, he shyly looked away. When he returned to her gaze, she was still looking! *Wow,* he thought, *she's incredible.*

The veteran nurses adored Dr. Afram, and they immediately sensed his attraction to Hiral. "She's not married, you know," one nurse coyly told him. "She's sweet, and amazingly smart—simply brilliant."

And sensual, thought Afram.

"Why don't you say something to her?" the nurse asked.

Afram quickly snapped back to reality, dismissed her question with a shake of his head, and continued his rounds with patients.

Days later, he saw Hiral again, and when their eyes met this time she smiled. Apparently, the nurses had meddled in Afram's love life, or absence thereof. Hiral was onto Afram; the nurses had told her he was interested.

Sensing an obligation to speak, Afram said "Hi." They spoke briefly. He asked her what she did at the hospital, even though he already knew. When the conversation ended, she handed him one of the nutrition pamphlets. He looked at it curiously. Walking away, he turned the pamphlet over and saw the handwritten words, "Kareem, call me sometime." She called him by his first name! *That was gutsy,* he thought. Afram respected Hiral for her boldness and immediately recognized there was something special about her.

Hiral and Afram's courtship was off to a brilliant start. They shared together whatever available time they had, and they became the darling couple of the hospital. Hiral was the only woman Afram ever met who made his heart melt. He let down his guard around her, taking off his superhero costume. They exchanged flirtatious glances and stares in the hospital throughout the day, and at night they filled each other with joy and completeness.

"How did we get here?" Afram asked one day.

"You've brought joy to my life, and you make me laugh and smile, and I feel free," Hiral answered. "You have a strong heart, Kareem," she added. With her head resting on his chest she could hear, feel, and connect with Kareem's strong heartbeat that Dr. Lloyd had helped him discover as a child.

Afram was very happy. He had a priceless love in Hiral, and she reciprocated that love, and more. He let his confident hospital façade down with her. To Hiral, the great Dr. Afram was just Kareem, the man she loved. They were committed to each other, and Afram's life became grounded in a way he'd never experienced. Hiral was there to comfort him when his surgical cases didn't go well, and to celebrate his success when they did.

Now many years moved away from New York and his mother, Afram had found for the first time something he cared about more than medicine and surgery. And unlike the jealous mistresses of the operating room and surgery that took and demanded so much and gave little in return, Hiral cared about Afram and gave him a type of comfort and inner peace he never found in his work. Hiral held the key to Afram's heart.

One night together, a phone call broke the silence and woke them both up. It was unusual for Afram's home phone to ring. Usually his pager would go off when the hospital needed him.

"Hello," Hiral answered. Afram sat up in bed.

"Yes, yes…oh, no…I, I see…. Yes—yes, yes, hold on. He's right here." Hiral was shaking as she slowly handed Afram the phone. It was the hospital—only this time the patient wasn't one of his. This time the patient was his mother, and the hospital was in New York.

The doctor told Afram that his mother had suffered a devastating stroke and had fallen. She had been found by a friend, and wasn't responsive. "It doesn't look good, sir," the doctor continued. "We're not sure…how much longer she'll hold on."

Afram and Hiral headed to New York on the next flight. All of Afram's composure and courage abandoned him. He was despondent.

Hiral and Afram stood together at Miriam's bedside. Her eyes closed peacefully, motionless. Afram was instantly brought to tears when he saw his mother in this condition.

He had last seen her only months earlier for Easter, and she had been vibrant and full of energy.

Afram was very familiar with that look she gave now—one of suspended animation, the brain and mind gone, the soul idle and trapped, simply waiting to be released by a body that was merely still holding on. He had seen that look in many of his patients before they died and he harvested their organs for transplantation.

Afram and Hiral watched and listened to the beeps on the monitor as Miriam's once-strong heart declined. The rate of heartbeats declined to forty, thirty, twenty, ten—and then no more. Silence. Right before their eyes, she was gone.

At his mother's funeral, Afram, holding back tears that never came for his father, eulogized his mother with a letter he read aloud.

"With every end, there's a new beginning," he said. "I wish we could still be together, Mom, but please know that we will always be together in spirit."

He paused to clear his throat.

"Mom, I want to thank you—and I want everyone here to know how much I appreciate all that you've done for me. You struggled to manage an unruly teenager when Dad died, and it was not easy—I know. I want to thank you today for what you did, and especially for three gifts you have given me in life. I can never repay you for them, but I will always treasure all three.

"Thank you for giving me *courage*. You left your home in Africa many years ago, seeking a better life. You had the courage to leave everything you knew and venture to a new land far away where you knew no one. Many people don't have the courage to do that. I'm glad that you had it.

"Thank you for giving me *strength*. You have tremendous strength. You were never idle, and you showed me the value of hard work. Because of your strength and your industry in a foreign land, working many hours at thankless jobs and sacrificing so much, you ensured that I could live a better life.

"Thank you for giving me *faith*. Do you remember when you told me I could be or do whatever I wanted in this country as long as I worked hard, had faith in God, and prayed? I will always remember your instructions well, and because of the faith you've given me in myself, I've been able to do many things in life.

"Lastly, Mom, I also want to thank you for your love. *All that I am or hope to be, I owe to you.*"

After his mother's death, Afram turned inward to his work, and Hiral was his constant support. Their love remained passionate and grew and matured over time. Dr. Afram became very busy with transplants. Often he would fly to procure organs and bring them back for recipients waiting for transplantation. He flew usually once or twice a week, much to the worry and concern of Hiral. Afram, however, enjoyed flying. He would even volunteer to go when he wasn't on call. Flying gave him a chance to literally step away from the world, and to think. He always believed his work was noble. Afram was off again to save the world.

He had learned years earlier that transplant surgery always happened at night, on weekends, and on holidays. It seemed that was when people were hurt. The transplant teams would land in the city, usually under the cloak of darkness. Trauma to the head and subsequent brain death was almost always the common denominator in all transplant donors.

Each story was always tragic. It was a suicide, a car accident, a fall, or sometimes a stroke. The young age of the victims troubled and fascinated Afram. The abruptness of trauma scared him. Afram would tell himself, "Almost every one of these patients who become organ donors left their home in the morning thinking everything was going to be okay—just a normal day, a routine day; *it's all going to be fine.*" Then just like that, an accident caused some head trauma that progressed to brain death—and that person became an organ donor candidate. Without the brain, the body will not survive—this is truth. The body may hold on for a time, but eventually it dies as well. There is an inextricable connection between the mind and the body.

The first transplant Dr. Afram did was a kidney transplant during his surgical residency in New York City. Later, when he did his first heart transplant, he was in awe. It was like being part of a miracle. The other surgical team harvested the organ, and he was on the team to implant the heart into the recipient. He remembered taking the cold heart out of the ice, holding it in his warm hands. It was a flaccid muscle with no activity and appeared incapable for the task that was now demanded. Afram's hands became cold and numb from the ice. He remembered performing the transplant operation with grace and precision. He meticulously attached the atrial chambers to the recipient, then sewed the vessels, the veins, and the arteries. When the transplanted heart warmed up and started to beat for that first time, Afram was filled with emotion, believing he was the privileged witness of a divine power at work.

Afram's work in transplant surgery always placed him on both sides of the continuum of life. At the donor's bedside, tragedy had taken away life. The circumstances created an opportunity so that a gift of life could be given out from that loss for the sake of someone else in need. The decision for the families was often hard. The finality signaled that hope for recovery had vanished. There was always sadness, grief, and loss. When the consent was given, it meant that the loved one was letting go and saying, "Okay, I'll give you up now—hopefully a part of you can continue to live in another person." It was an incredible gift.

At the recipient's bedside, joy, anxiety, and anticipation would be running high. The patient had a bad heart, was often very sick, and was living an uncomfortable life facing death in a matter of months, weeks, or sometimes days. The new heart, they hoped, would bring new life. These patients felt themselves at the edge of life, and they were very familiar with their mortality, wasting never a moment with petty things. The operation and new heart gave them a new lease on life—and Afram was part of making that possible.

When heart transplant surgery goes well, the patients are literally walking miracles, and Afram thought that he had made it happen. Afram once met a patient in Chicago with a transplanted heart as well as both lungs transplanted. After thirty years he was still going strong and extremely active. He was the embodiment of what one person's gift could do. In a special celebration, he was honored by the transplant community, like a celebrity. His children and grandchildren were there to be a part of it. It was a beautiful moment.

These thoughts occupied Afram as he flew around the country doing his work. He felt a great sense of satisfaction. He felt like a broker of the gift of life.

On one occasion he arrived with his team at a hospital in Iowa to harvest a heart. The patient was a twenty-four-year-old trauma victim with a head injury in an accident involving alcohol. It was a sad case.

Afram conducted his usual checklist. He searched the donor patient's chart to make sure the consent form for donating organs was in place. He reviewed the echocardiogram that showed the pictures of the heart. He made sure there was a brain death notification certified by two physicians. Finally, he ensured that the donor's blood type matched that of the recipient back at his home hospital in Minnesota.

Many of these operations involved multiple teams, and since the transplant world was so small, it was common to have minireunions in different cities with various other transplant surgeons and teams. There was the liver team, the kidney and pancreas team, and—on rare occasions—a small bowel team. Afram met with his community of surgeons in random hospitals at night, on holidays, and usually on weekends to do the work of transplantation. All teams competed for the limited real estate at the operating room table, harvesting and procuring organs to transport them back to their respective home institutions for desperately ill and waiting patients on the other side.

Transplant was a coordinated team effort. As the head of the heart team, Afram dictated the timing and conduct of the entire operation for all the teams, since the heart was always the first organ to be removed before any other. Each team made their calls back to the home institution to make sure their recipient was prepared and ready.

Communication was key. Monitoring the blood pressure of the donor patient was essential, as was talking with the anesthesiologist and with the other teams. Teamwork was everything.

Finally, after all the calls were made and the recipient teams were ready, and transportation was arranged to go back home, Afram would make the critical decision on the time to cross-clamp the aorta and stop the flow of blood through the major vessel that left the heart to carry blood throughout the entire body.

Once this critical action was performed, there was no turning back. The clock started to tick, and there wasn't a moment to lose or a second to waste; the organs began to die once the cross clamp was placed.

All the organs were infused with a cold preservative and packed on ice. Once the blood stopped flowing to the organs, they were at risk until the organs were transplanted into a new body and life-giving blood was restored to each organ in their new recipients. For the heart, the donor-to-recipient time window was usually four hours.

"Okay, the heart is out," Afram confirmed on that day in the hospital in Iowa. He held the organ close to his chest, just as he'd done hundreds of times before, and took the precious heart to the back operating room table. With quick movements, the heart was packaged in plastic bags and containers and placed in an ice-filled cooler labeled HEART ORGAN FOR HUMAN TRANSPLANT.

He checked his watch and confirmed the time of cross-clamp.

"Is the ambulance waiting?" he asked. "Make sure the pilots know we're on our way." On one occasion, Afram and his team had gone down to the ambulance bay with harvested lungs in tow, and there was no transportation to the airport! They waited with an organ on ice for a half hour with no ride. Fortunately everything worked out well, but it impressed upon Afram to never take logistics for granted. Now he *always* checked and double-checked every detail.

Afram looked at his watch. *Thirty-five minutes so far.*

The team arrived at the airport after driving through downtown Iowa City from the hospital with ambulance lights flashing and sirens blaring.

"Gentlemen, how are things?" Afram asked the pilots.

"Good, sir," the pilot answered.

"What's our flight time?"

"About an hour."

Afram mentally calculated—thirty-five minutes already gone, plus an hour in flight, then another half hour on the ground—just over two hours total.

"Great," he finally said. "That will give our team back home plenty of time. How's our weather for the flight back?"

"Looks like mostly clear skies, with some weather that we'll avoid in southern Minnesota," the pilot answered.

Afram had also learned to ask about such things. Minnesota was known for its severe weather, especially in winter. Flying could be hazardous, dangerous, in some cases lethal. A few years ago an entire transplant team was lost when their flight went down in a storm. It was an absolute tragedy, and the entire transplant community mourned the great loss to society. On that fateful flight, in one accident, a collective sixty years of superspecialized clinical experience was lost.

Afram's flight back was smooth, and they landed just over an hour later. "Thank you, gentlemen, always a pleasure," Afram said.

The pilots waved back, and one of them called out, "Good luck, sir! We'll see you next time."

Back in the ambulance, and en route back to the hospital and the recipient team, Afram routinely placed two calls. One call was to the recipient team, alerting them to the status of their travel. The next call was to Hiral, to let her know he was back home and safe.

"Hi, honey, it's me!" Afram said. "Everything went well. I'm on my way back to the hospital and should be home soon. The other team will be doing the transplant this time."

There was silence on the other end of the line.

"Is everything all right?" Afram asked.

Hiral finally answered, "We need to talk when you get home."

"Talk about what?" Afram asked, sensing her ominous tone.

"It's not something we can discuss over the phone," she answered.

"You're making me worried. Is everything okay?"

"I can't talk about it right now," Hiral responded. "Just wait until you get home."

Afram's heart sank. Hiral and Afram had had their differences over the years, but they were *always* able to talk over the phone. Her hesitance was very unusual—and Afram could think of nothing else until he made it home.

When he came through the door, all the lights were off except in the bedroom.

"Hiral?" Afram called.

"I'm in the bedroom," she answered. Afram found her quietly sitting on the bed. He sat beside her and held her hand tenderly.

"What's wrong?" he asked. "You look like you've been crying, and you're sitting here in a dark house. What happened today, and why are you so upset?" he asked again.

"Do you love me?" she asked.

Taken aback, Afram sensed the question was a trick. "What do you mean?"

"I need to know. Do you love me?" she asked again.

"Of course I do. What's this all about?"

"I—I was very excited today. I found out some wonderful news, and I couldn't wait to share with you."

Afram raised his eyebrows in anticipation and squeezed her hand.

Hiral continued, "But I also found out some news that was very upsetting." She pulled an envelope from her side and held it close to her heart. Afram stared at her, then at the envelope she held tightly.

"What's that?"

"It's a letter addressed to you, and I answered a call from your unit at the Minnesota Armory today. They called to find out if you received this letter."

"Well, let's open it," he said, moving closer to her.

"Before I give you this letter, I have something to tell you," she stated. "I'm pregnant, Kareem. We're going to have a baby."

Really! That's wonderful! That's great news, I'm so happy." Afram embraced Hiral, crushing the letter as they hugged. He sensed that she wasn't squeezing back, and he withdrew.

"What's wrong?" he asked. "Aren't you happy?"

"Of course. Of course I am. It's just that—" With tears in her eyes, she extended to Afram the now-crumpled letter.

"What does it say?" he asked. "Do you know what the Armory wanted? Is it about my drill next weekend?"

"No—it's not about your drill weekend," she told him. "Open it, just open it!"

Afram ripped open the letter, which was addressed from the U.S. Navy Reserve. He unfolded the documents and scanned quickly. "Commander Kareem Afram, Medical Corps, US Navy Reserve...WHEN DIRECTED BY REPORTING SENIOR, DETACH FOR ASSIGNMENT IN SUPPORT OF OVERSEAS CONTINGENCY OPERATIONS AFGHANISTAN."

Afram was speechless and numb. A well of emotions filled him. In a very short time he'd lost his mother, learned he would be a father, and now discovered he was being deployed to Afghanistan.

Afram had joined the Navy reserves years earlier after the tragedy of 9/11. He was a surgical resident in New York City and watched, from the rooftop of his hospital in real time, the Twin Towers come crashing down, changing his beloved New York City skyline forever. His hospital scrambled and prepared to accept casualties, but very few patients came— there were no survivors. Afram sensed a void and felt helpless, like many other physicians in the city. He wanted to help, but couldn't.

When the war in Iraq started, he saw his opportunity. Men and women would be injured, and he knew he could help. Afram felt that service in the Navy was a way to give back to the country that had provided so many opportunities to his parents and himself. Afram chose the Navy because he knew he would travel, it was exciting, and he thought they had the best uniforms.

Subconsciously, Afram also knew his success in the Navy was redemptive and would prove himself to be better than his father, Kwame. As a child, his father, Kwame, had failed to last on the fishing boat, but now in the Navy Afram would succeed. Indeed, when Afram initially joined the Navy, he welcomed the adventure, looked forward to deployment, and even enjoyed his brief time out to sea. He was a single, young, carefree surgeon living only for himself. But that was before Hiral came into his life, before the death of his mother—and before he was to become a father.

His weekend drills and temporary assignments were always local and of little intrusion on the idyllic life he'd created with Hiral. Now things were much different. He'd found the love of his life, and he had a child on the way.

Afram realized the danger of this assignment in the desert and sensed his mortality. He knew what he had to do.

A week later, Hiral and Afram were married in the St. Paul City Hall. Afram's parents were now gone, and Hiral's parents couldn't travel from India in time. Hiral and Afram celebrated the event with a small dinner party with close friends. They enjoyed the moment, and didn't share with anyone the news about their baby on the way—at least not yet.

PART II

To Serve

◇

Afghanistan

"INBOUND, INBOUND, CATEGORY ALPHA, Category Alpha," the Charlie Company Marine corporal announced. "Cat-A casualty, ten minutes out!"

Afram and his medical unit, Echo Surgical Company, had just landed at the Forward Operating Base Musa Kala—a.k.a. FOB MK. The small austere base was ground zero for Marine casualties. It was nestled in the Sangin Valley of Helmand Province in southwest Afghanistan. The Marines were engaged in heavy firefights throughout the region, and FOB MK was the closest base with medical capability.

Echo Surgical Company was transported to FOB MK in a CH-53 Sea Stallion helicopter, the largest and heaviest of the Marine Corps aircraft. Afram and his unit looked out across the desert landscape as they approached the base. *Nothing around for miles*, Afram thought.

Unlike the slick jets Afram enjoyed for his transplant work back home, these military helicopters made Afram very anxious. The old aircraft shook violently. Oil and grease leaked from everywhere, and Afram sat in a puddle of grease en route to FOB MK.

"Welcome to FOB MK, sir," the corporal said. "Sir, you can all leave your bags at the flight line—we have a Cat-A inbound. Should be here in eight minutes!"

"How was your flight in, sir?" the corporal asked.

"Good," Afram said reluctantly.

"Well, sir, we're happy you guys are all here," the corporal said excitedly, "because that means we get to go home! As you know, sir, this is a bad neighborhood. Just to our south is the Pakistan border, and to the west is the Iranian border. We've been taking heavy casualties for months securing this region."

Afram and his team had arrived in Afghanistan two weeks earlier, after eight weeks of training stateside. It was an ordeal to finally get to FOB MK, and it felt surreal to Afram. Echo Surgical Company had five surgeons and almost two hundred medical personnel distributed throughout the Helmand and Nimroz provinces to medically support the fighting U.S. Marines. Afram, two other surgeons, and a team of thirty-five others—including emergency room doctors, nurses, physician's assistants, and Navy hospital corpsmen—were sent to FOB MK because it was the busiest base for casualties.

"Sir, you guys can leave your weapons in our armory," the corporal instructed. "I know you've been carrying them around all this time, but they'll be safe in our STP/FRSS." This was Shock Trauma Platoon/Forward Resuscitative Surgical System—the main tent where the medical team worked. There was space for triage of patients, stretchers, and supplies, and the FRSS part of the tent system had two ORs with basic supplies.

"That's great news!" Afram said. Everyone had been issued weapons, and each officer had two firearms—a rifle and a pistol. Afram carried his M4 rifle and M9 pistol everywhere. Like the other physicians, he was initially uncomfortable with them. But after an indoctrination and training for eight weeks with the Marines, plus a sobering appreciation that the enemy didn't spare doctors from harm, Afram grew to appreciate and almost love his weapons, and became "surgically" skilled in handling them. Afram even adopted the Marines' custom of assigning a female name to his weapons. He named his M4 rifle Tonya, while his M9 pistol was Sonia.

"Cat-A one minute away!" yelled the corporal. The sound of the DUSTOFF helicopter could now be heard. DUSTOFF was an acronym for Dedicated Unhesitating Service to Our Fighting Forces. As their name implied, besides always raising a cloud of dust when they took off and landed, these helicopter aircraft never hesitated to fly into enemy hell to rescue injured Marines. They were badass. Over time, Afram could identify what helicopter was approaching FOB MK by their sound alone.

Anxiety now filled everyone on the new team. Category A casualties were the most serious of injuries and usually were life-threatening. Almost all casualties brought to FOB MK were Cat-As.

Unfortunately, Afram had already witnessed his first combat death in Afghanistan at the larger hospital one week prior. It was a British soldier with a lethal gunshot wound to the pelvis. Nothing, however, would prepare him and the team for what was to come.

"Go, go, go!" The litter bearers ran into the plume of dust as the helicopter landed with the injured Marine. The team, including Afram, scurried to the wall around the STP for shelter from the cloud of blinding sand-dust that now covered the entry to the STP/FRSS.

"Eighteen-year-old Marine, IED victim," the DUSTOFF crew reported. "Two lower extremity injuries and left hand injury. Blood pressure is seventy-over-palp with a weak pulse. We couldn't get an IV line in him." As the crew finished the report, the Marine emerged from the dust cloud on the stretcher with the corpsmen carrying him to the threshold of the STP.

About 95 percent of all injuries in Afghanistan were caused by an Improvised Explosive Device (IED)—the enemy's weapon of choice, because it was cheap, effective, and easy to use. Afram and Echo Surgical Company had learned all about IEDs stateside, during their training with the Marines.

The look on the Marine's face was unforgettable, and that first vision haunted Afram forever. He was only a kid. He was a ghost color, with sunken eyes rolled back, his mouth opened slightly, his lips dry, and dirt covering every inch of his body. What struck Afram above all was the Marine's lower body. He had no legs—just blood-soaked, dirt-soiled shreds of uniform with charred muscle and tendons dangling off bone. The Marine slowly waved his bruised right arm as if reaching for something only he could see. His left hand was missing—only a bloody stump was present, with dirty bandages suppressing the bleeding.

The experienced Charlie Surgical Company went to work on the Marine after they brought him into the STP. They cut off his clothes, set up an IV, and prepared him for surgery.

Afram was now the uninitiated. He'd seen and experienced much in the sterile, controlled settings of hospitals stateside. This was different. He was in a tent in the middle of the desert, with a patient who'd been blown up to pieces. Nothing he'd experienced before compared to this.

Afram's heart wrenched. The young Marine was in shock—his eyes screamed despair, pain, and horror. He was the picture of death. Afram and the Echo surgical team were also in shock. The team quickly moved the Marine into the FRSS operating room. The Charlie Company team worked with skill, adeptness, precision, and teamwork. Afram and his Echo surgical team, all fully trained health professionals, were completely lost, some holding back dry heaves from the sight of the injured Marine.

Afram quickly realized the only thing keeping the Marine alive were the two small tourniquets wrapped around his thighs, up high by the groin. Only these two straps kept the Marine from completely bleeding to death. Afram would learn later that Marines actually put tourniquets on *before* they went on a mission. Their philosophy was not *if*, but rather *when* they would be injured by an IED. Afram always respected the Marines, but witnessing this young man—and appreciating the mental fortitude he and his fellow Marines had to possess each day to step out beyond the wire on patrol and face the risks of IEDs—increased Afram's respect for them all the more. Here was either the greatest example of courage, or something just plain crazy, Afram concluded.

"We need blood in here," announced the Charlie Company anesthesiologist. The OR was dusty and primitive compared to those back in the States, or even those at the larger bases. At FOB MK, only the basic essentials were available—nothing fancy. The *only* objective here was to save lives.

"You guys should scrub in," one of the Charlie Company surgeons said to Afram and the other surgeon from Echo Company. "No better way to get started."

Afram washed his hands with the pump water and donned a gown.

The room was painfully hot. Afram moved with an uncommon trepidation. He was in unfamiliar territory. There was nothing elegant about the case.

"Let's get more water over here," ordered the surgeon from Charlie Company. The seasoned members of Charlie Surgical Company prepared the Marine's extremities for surgery. The corpsmen held the Marine's destroyed stumps, all that were left of his legs, and washed them as best they could as the mass of bleeding skin, muscle, and shattered bone slipped between their hands. They pulled leaves, sand, rocks, and mud from fibers of charred and burnt muscle and tendon. Trauma shears were used to cut away the dead tissue, in much the same way as a butcher cutting fat from a side of beef.

The Marine had lost everything below the knees. Most of his thighs on both sides were destroyed. His genitalia were bruised and the scrotum cut open. "Just look for the major vessels," the Charlie Company surgeon instructed. "We want to tie off the femoral artery and vein."

Even for Afram, an anatomical master, it was a challenge to find vessels in a bed of charred flesh and destroyed landmarks, where everything bled. *Hamburger surgery,* Afram thought. Blood soaked the wooden tent floor as it dripped from the stretcher.

Afram's gown was now saturated in sweat, blood, and the Marine's burnt muscle and dead tissue. As Afram shifted his weight while he worked, his boots stuck to the floor from the paste made of blood, sweat, and sand.

It was beyond hot. Sweat ran down Afram's back and down his legs. He also saw sweat pouring off the forehead and nose of the Charlie Company surgeon, and dripping directly into the Marine's wound.

Surgical technique and everything Afram knew of surgical etiquette was thrown out the window.

"We need more blood!" the anesthesiologist called again.

Conspiring against Afram were the desert heat, the lung-filling sand-dust, dehydration, a bumpy CH-53 helo ride, and the bloody scene. He grew wobbly and short of breath, and felt faint. His tall, slender, erect superhero frame was now limp from the kryptonite of heat, anguish, and physical and emotional exhaustion.

"We need the walking blood bank," the anesthesiologist ordered. As soon as a Cat-A trauma victim was inbound, dozens of Marines on the base would come to the medical STP/FRSS tents and wait to give their blood to their fallen brethren. Every Marine knew his blood type, and a rotation system for donors ensured a fresh supply of available donors. On this occasion, ten Marines had come to medical to donate A-positive blood type for the injured victim.

Afram worked on what was left of the Marine's stump. "Yes, just like that," the Charlie Company surgeon confirmed. "We need to remove as much of the dead tissue as possible." This wasn't heart surgery, but as he worked, Afram—always a great surgeon at heart—recited to himself the top three rules of trauma surgery: *1) Stop the bleeding. 2) Stop the bleeding. 3) Stop the bleeding!*

There were four surgeons working on the young Marine, two on each extremity. "How long have we been working?" the Charlie Company surgeon asked.

"Fifty minutes," a nurse answered, as she documented vitals.

"We try and aim for under an hour with these cases," the Charlie Company surgeon said. "We've learned—much longer than that, and it's a losing battle. They just keep bleeding, the blood stops clotting, and the game's over. Our objective is strictly damage control—nothing definitive. We're here to stop the bleeding, cut away as much of the dead tissue as we can, and get the Marine transferred to a higher echelon of care as soon as possible."

The other Charlie Company surgeon added, "This is the first operation of about fifty or more this young guy will have before all is said and done. Besides, we have to move quickly, because it's only a matter of time before the next Cat-A Marine comes through our STP and we have to be ready."

Afram carefully recorded the wise words of these experienced surgeons. He knew that in only two days, the Charlie team would be shipping out, turnover would be done, and Afram and his Echo Surgical Company colleagues would be on their own.

"That's the fifteenth unit of blood, sir," anesthesia reported.

Fifteen units of blood, Afram thought. *Incredible!* He would learn later that the Marine received more than forty additional units of blood in subsequent operations at the next echelons of care, before he ever left Afghanistan and headed back to the States.

"Okay, let's get him packaged up," the Charlie Company surgeon ordered. "Call DUSTOFF and let them know we're ready for Evac in ten minutes!"

"Thanks for taking us through this," Afram said gratefully to the Charlie Company surgeons.

"Not a problem," one of the surgeons said. "Our pleasure! You guys are essentially in charge now. What people don't realize back home is that out here in the desert of Afghanistan, all that stuff you guys learn in textbooks and do in the hospitals back home gets tossed right out!"

"Absolutely," added the other surgeon. "War and being a combat trauma surgeon makes you extremely creative."

Indeed, Afram would learn about the many advances made in the desert that weren't known or taught back home. Combat surgeons learned decisively how lives were saved through tourniquets, addressing bleeding before anything else, and using the walking blood bank to deliver whole fresh blood to trauma victims instead of banked blood. These things were responsible for the low mortality over the past decade of war, and for an improved long-term picture for young people with devastating injuries. Still, Afram couldn't imagine what life was like for those wounded warriors.

The injured Marine was transported to the Role III echelon of care, to a larger base with more capability and hard-structured operating rooms with far better facilities. After surgery there, he was transported to a large Role IV base in Europe. Ultimately the Marine made the trip back home to be taken care of at one of the major medical centers in the States that was designated a Role V Military Treatment Facility. Typically, injured Marines would be back to the States within thirty-six to seventy-two hours after being injured. This was a testament to the military's incredible logistics and a dedicated team of professional military personnel.

FOB MK was a Role II base. After injured Marines received Role I point-of-injury care from corpsmen in the field, Afram and his team of Echo Surgical Company were next in line to care for these wounded.

"Two more Cat-Alphas inbound—Cat-Alpha times two inbound," the corporal yelled.

"No rest for you guys," a Charlie Company surgeon chuckled. "Welcome to FOB MK."

"What's coming in?" Afram asked.

Two more Marines with IED injuries were arriving with below-knee amputations.

In less than thirty-six hours after arriving at FOB MK, Echo Surgical Company treated five Category Alpha patients, with fifteen injured extremities. The patients were all Marines blown up by IEDs. All these wounded warriors were missing legs, arms, or hands, and one Marine had lost both arms and legs as well as his testicles. The team saved them all.

The process was always the same. Stop the bleeding, activate the walking blood bank, stabilize the Marine, work very quickly, and transfer the patient to a higher echelon of care.

The novel shock of the first couple of Cat-Alpha cases wore off for Afram and for most of the Echo Surgical Company. There was no time to process the reality that greeted them with each injury.

Afram quickly erected a protective shell of indifference around himself to maintain his composure, to keep from feeling emotion, and to continue coping with the sight of blown-up young Marines. He closed his heart to feelings. Feelings had no business in this place, he concluded; feelings would never help him here in the desert. It was a harsh and hostile environment where pain, death, and destruction were frequent visitors.

Echo Surgical Company ceremoniously said farewell to Charlie Surgical Company, and they watched with envy as the team departed on the CH 53 helicopter heading for home. Their departure was bittersweet; Afram and his Echo surgical team faced the sobering reality that they were here for good until their relief came in eight months.

As Charlie Company's helo departed and disappeared over the Afghan horizon, Echo Company heard, "Cat-Alpha—times two, inbound five minutes out!"

The two Marines who came in were victims of sniper gunshot wounds. The bullets pierced their extremities and flanks that were unprotected by body armor. One Marine was unstable and clearly had a serious abdominal injury. Afram and one of the other Echo Surgical Company surgeons scrubbed in to take care of the unstable Marine, while the orthopedic surgeon cared for the other injured Marine.

Afram and the rookie Echo Surgical Company team moved slowly and awkwardly, but managed to get the Marine on the operating room table. Afram and the other surgeon made an incision over the Marine's belly, and once the abdominal cavity was entered, blood poured out of the Marine and onto the stretcher and the surgeons' legs. "Lap sponges! Quick, we need lap sponges!" Afram ordered. "Let's pack the abdomen," he said, as he shoved surgical sponges into the belly in an attempt to dam up the hemorrhage and keep the blood in the Marine's body.

Andre Chester was the other Echo Company surgeon working with Afram. "I can see the injury," Chester said, as Afram held retraction for him. "Looks like the bullet pierced the flank and pelvis and traveled across the abdomen. There are several small and large intestine injuries, plus a shattered gallbladder, and the liver is injured as well."

Commander Andre Chester was an outstanding technical general surgeon with sound operative judgment. He was a Naval Academy graduate and planned on staying in the Navy forever. His father served in Vietnam as a decorated A-4 naval pilot, while his grandfather flew naval air strikes as an officer in the Korean War; both men were also graduates of the Naval Academy. Chester was jokingly seen as the black sheep in the family because he became a doctor instead of a pilot.

"His blood pressure's low!" Afram announced. "Give him more blood."

"The seventh unit is going in right now," the anesthesiologist responded.

"We'll give you guys a chance to catch up," Afram said. "He needs to be resuscitated." Chester and Afram both had their hands in the Marine's abdomen, holding pressure on the injuries, while containing the bleeding liver. The surgeons worked well together, providing tension and countertension as they dissected through the viscera of the abdomen. They repaired the holes in the intestine, resected the shattered gallbladder, repaired the bleeding vessels, and packed the injured liver to contain the hemorrhage.

An hour had passed when Chester announced, "Looks like things are under control here." Afram agreed.

As they finished, Peter Levine, the Echo Company orthopedic surgeon, came in to check on the team's progress. "The injuries are stable," he reported. "If you guys are done here, we can arrange for DUSTOFF to transport both Marines together to the Role III hospital."

Lieutenant Commander Peter Levine was truly a seasoned veteran. He was a brilliant young orthopedic surgeon and medical officer who recently completed his orthopedic surgery residency. He joined the Navy's ROTC program while at Harvard, and although he was only a lieutenant commander, Levine had deployed as a general medical officer more times than any other officer in Echo Company. This was his fourth deployment, of two each in Iraq and Afghanistan.

After the patients were transferred, the exhausted Afram, Levine, and Chester retired to their shared tent. The Echo Surgical Company's introduction to FOB MK had been chaotic, and none of the officers had unpacked their bags since arriving at the base. Their uniforms were saturated in blood and sweat made heavy by the Afghan desert-dust that settled in.

The days became a blur. In a very short time, the surgeons graduated from novice to seasoned combat surgeons, and they worked well together as a surgical unit. With each subsequent trauma case, the Echo Surgical Company rookie team moved closer to equaling the varsity performers of their Charlie Company predecessors.

FOB MK was extremely austere. There was no plumbing, and Afram had already learned how to use the piss tubes and wag bags. Deep holes were dug, and PVC tubing inserted into the ground to collect urine in the tubes. Everyone on base captured their feces in plastic "wag bags" that were collected and ultimately burned.

Communication back home was sporadic and unpredictable. Afram managed to speak briefly to Hiral only a couple of times, and long enough to find out the wonderful news that Hiral's latest ultrasound confirmed a healthy baby boy was growing in her womb. Afram shared this excitement with his fellow tent mates. Levine was twice divorced without children; Chester was happily married with four young kids.

The food at FOB MK was awful, and the heat—averaging 120 degrees Fahrenheit—was unbearable.

When two days passed without a casualty, the short break from trauma provided Afram with a chance to think. On a hard cot in his shared tent, he stared at the roof of the canvas and nylon structure. The air contained a hint of burning wag bags mixed with Afghan sand-dust.

Sharing his constant thoughts of Hiral were his thoughts about his unborn child, as he tried to stifle the frustration of knowing he wouldn't be there to see his son born.

Afram closed his eyes. He took in a breath and coughed. He choked on the sand-dust that was ubiquitous and attached to everything, right down to the cells of his lungs. He coughed again and released a sigh. *It's going to be a long eight months.*

He prayed for his time to go by fast.

◇

The Tent

FIVE MONTHS HAD PASSED SINCE ECHO SURGICAL Company arrived at FOB MK and said farewell to Charlie Company.

Become comfortable with being uncomfortable, Afram thought as he tossed and turned on his cot in his shared tent. He scratched his head violently, sensing that the mouse which had previously taunted him was back in the cot with him and crawling over his head. Finally, finding a position of brief comfort, he smiled in his sleep.

His brief moment of happiness soon ended with sound of the dreaded trauma bell. After five months at FOB MK, Afram could sleep through the loud bickering of Chester and Levine, an irritating mouse, and the roar of the helicopters— even the loudest Ospreys, which shook the entire base and rattled his flimsy tent and cot. But no one could sleep through the trauma bell's distinctive sound.

"Wake your asses up…Wake your Goddamn asses up!" Corporal Smalls yelled, ringing the trauma bell incessantly and waking everyone up from pillow quarters. He yelled again, "Cat-Alpha inbound!"

It was zero-dark-thirty, and Corporal Smalls was on night duty. His job was to wake up the surgical team day or night whenever a casualty was inbound, and he took his responsibility seriously.

Smalls was a scrappy kid from Tulsa, Oklahoma, who proudly stated, "I have a PHD—Plain-ass High-school Diploma!" The son of a single mom, Smalls chose to join the Marines over the other option offered by the judge: going to jail for parole violation.

Corporal Smalls had become an expert marksman and fine infantryman. He was perturbed that now he was assigned to babysit the "sissy Navy medical team" instead of fighting with his fellow Marine brothers outside the wire.

"What do we have, corporal?" Afram asked, yawning as they entered the STP/FRSS.

"Sir, we have a Cat-Alpha Marine who fell down a ninety-foot well while on patrol," he answered.

"Ninety feet?" Afram asked in disbelief. "Are there wells in this area of the desert?"

"Affirmative, sir, that was the report. Lieutenant Ryzik told me to wake everyone up. He thinks the injuries could be bad because of the mechanism."

Lieutenant Ryzik was the young emergency medicine doctor on the Echo surgical team. He was fresh out of residency, and an eager beaver. He had graduated from Georgetown undergrad and signed up for the Navy's Health Professions Scholarship Program to help pay for medical school at Duke. Ryzik was green; this was his first deployment and first opportunity to be in charge of anything. He was responsible for the initial assessment of all patients who entered the STP. Now even after five months at FOB MK, he was still overly cautious, sometimes to a fault.

The Afghan desert and the stars in the night sky laughed and winked at the tired team running back and forth to empty their bladders in the piss tubes. All of Echo Surgical Company's medical team was now assembled and waiting in the STP area of the tent for the Cat-Alpha. It was common to have all hands on deck when a trauma arrived, since so much was needed from everyone.

"Cat-Alpha arriving," Corporal Smalls announced.

The corpsman ran out into the dust plume and darkness to retrieve yet another Cat-Alpha. The Marine arrived in the STP, fully alert, talking and looking around—in stark contrast to the usual Cat-Alphas.

"Check his vitals, let's get his uniform off," Ryzik ordered.

Until a patient definitively needed surgery, Lieutenant Ryzik was in charge. The surgeons—Afram, Levine, and Chester—impatiently looked over the shoulders of the busy Echo surgical team attempting to assess the Marine's injuries.

"Okay, blood pressure one-thirty over seventy," the nurse reported. "Heart rate is eighty-five, and his pulse oximetry is 100 percent. He's moving all extremities, fully awake, and completely stable."

"He looks more like a Cat-Zulu," Levine observed, catching the opposite end of the military alphabet from alpha. After a fourth deployment, Levine was a master of sarcasm and cynicism. "It doesn't look like anything's broken," he added.

"What's your name, Marine?" Levine asked as he approached the stretcher.

"Ah—ah, my name is Modesto Ruiz. Private Modesto Ruiz, sir."

"Are you having any pain anywhere?"

"No—no sir. Ah, actually, my nose hurts, sir."

"Your nose?"

"Ah—yes sir, my nose!" the Marine repeated.

"Private Ruiz, tell me what happened to you."

"Well sir, I—I was on patrol, and I saw a light in the desert, and it was traveling toward me at the speed of Mach holy shit, sir—sorry, sir. I tried to move out of the way, and fell down a ditch, sir."

"A ditch? We were told you fell down a well. How deep was this ditch?"

"Ah, sir, it was seven, maybe nine feet."

"Did you report this to your squadron leader?"

"Yes, sir."

"Clearly there was a breakdown in communication," Levine assessed, and he began a brief lecture. "When I was on my last deployment, a Marine colonel told me that Marines must do three things—Marines have to shoot, Marines have to move, and Marines have to communicate. This colonel said no one on the planet moves better or shoots better than a United States Marine. Communication, however is sometimes a problem. And it's the one thing that, if done ineffectively, leads to the most trouble."

"Yes sir—you're right sir," the Marine agreed.

"Of course I'm right," Levine said. "I hope your nose gets better," he added, as he turned to Lieutenant Ryzik. "Lieutenant Ryzik is going to take very, very, very good care of you."

As he walked out of the STP, Levine mumbled, "Everybody has a right to be stupid, but some people abuse the privilege. I'm going back to bed."

A few hours after the false alarm, the sunrise cast a hazy light on the STP/FRSS. It was a Sunday morning, and usually the Echo surgical team had an easy day on Sunday. Afram and Commander Chester would go to Catholic Mass. Afram had stopped going to Mass years ago in the States, but here in the desert he found that attending the service helped him unwind. Afram bonded with Chester, who was very spiritual and at times evangelical.

Chaplains visited FOB MK infrequently, usually only twice a month, unlike the larger bases that had services almost daily. Still, FOB MK was fortunate to get bimonthly visits from the chaplains, and Afram and Chester seized the opportunity on every occasion.

On a base with three hundred individuals, attendance at Mass seemed unusually low, from Afram's perspective. On this Sunday there were only seven people present, including Afram, Chester, and the chaplain. Afram and Chester were usually the only two people from the Echo Surgical Company's thirty-five-member medical team who attended regularly.

Afram, Levine, and Chester were growing weary and more indifferent over their five months together. The surgeons had performed more than a hundred surgical cases, with three times that many injured extremities. Afram was continually humbled by the cases. In the week before the chaplain arrived for this Sunday's Mass, Afram had lost another Marine on the OR table from a gunshot wound to the chest. The bullet had transected the great vessels leaving the heart, and the Marine had no signs of life on arrival. But the team did everything they could, and Afram opened the Marine's chest and massaged his heart while the team poured blood into the young man. But nothing helped. It was a futile effort, and the blood simply poured out of the holes of the Marine's wounds. Afram learned that some injuries just outmatched his skills, and some injuries could never be fixed.

The patient was a *hero*. That was the name given to Marines killed in action.

After all the months of harsh living, poor food, and devastating casualties, Echo Surgical Company's morale was low. Afram's heart remained closed to emotion, so that he could cope with the constant carnage he saw almost daily. Although the team was more than halfway done with the deployment, the end still seemed very far away; they felt like they would never get home.

Afram and Chester welcomed spending time with the chaplain and having Mass. It was a brief spiritual escape from their harsh reality of combat, injury, and death.

The reading for the Mass was from First Corinthians, with a timely message to all seven in attendance. The chaplain admonished them to pray for opportunities to spread the good word of the Lord Jesus Christ, and to pray for wisdom concerning when to spread the word and with whom. Afram left the service inspired and with a lifted spirit.

The Mass services were always an event Afram looked forward to with enthusiasm, and on this occasion he went back to his tent to write a love letter to Hiral and to his unborn son. Hiral was due to deliver in just four weeks. Afram couldn't believe so much time had passed since Hiral shared with him the wonderful news about expecting their child.

The surgeons had become close over the months—mostly out of necessity. They had no choice. There could not have been three more different individuals assembled together in such close proximity.

Afram was moderate, calculated and cool, a "doctor elegant."

Peter Levine was a savvy, seasoned character who accepted no nonsense, and who carried heavy emotional scars from war and divorce. Levine graduated *summa cum laude* from Johns Hopkins Medical School. He had wit, and would proudly say, "I have the brains and sarcasm of a Jewish New Yorker, even though I grew up in Boston. I'm the best of both worlds." His views on the world were as liberal as the insults he dished out regularly with colorful expletives. Afram teased Levine about the Red Sox and claimed to be a Yankees fan, though he couldn't name three Yankees to save his life. But he always enjoyed stirring up Levine's emotions. He was easy to provoke.

Levine and Chester were always engaged in some conflict or debate. Levine was a self-proclaimed expert in military history, and he constantly quizzed Chester, the Naval Academy grad, about military facts and war trivia. There were personal attacks as well. Levine once walked into the tent and was greeted by an awful stench from Chester's unwashed clothes. He then asked, "Did the Maytag man come by when your dad was away and break your mother's heart? Your clothes haven't been washed in weeks, dude. It's unbelievable!" All three men erupted in laughter. Levine kept everyone's spirit up with his humor, stories, and sharp tongue.

Andre Chester grew up in Richmond, Virginia, and could trace his ancestry all the way back to Civil War days, though he never told Afram or Levine which side his family fought on. After the Naval Academy, he went to medical school at Vanderbilt after failing to qualify to fly jets, and he talked about hunting religiously.

During his stateside training, he had been asked to serve on an important staging committee to help assist nurses and medical reserve officers in their transition for deployment. In reply, Chester—who was a student of John Stuart Mill and made constant references to *The Federalist Papers*—offered this response: "Only two good things ever came out of committee work: the King James Bible and the U.S. Constitution. I don't think we can top that in any damn staging committee work. So I'm not interested."

Both Chester and Levine were surprised to learn that Afram had a Catholic background and attended Catholic school.

Afram bragged about his heart cases and poked fun at Levine. He told him once, "You operate like an orthopedic surgeon!" This was an obvious slight, coming from a heart surgeon.

Afram, Chester, and Levine each supported each other and attempted to create comfort out of a very difficult time.

Afram hung a picture of Hiral above his cot. He also enjoyed reading books that had been donated to the USO; he kept a stack of them in his tent. From one book he prized, the *Meditations* of Marcus Aurelius, came a passage that was Afram's favorite: "Dwell on the beauty of life, watch the stars, and see yourself running with them.... You have power over your mind—not outside events. Realize this, and you will find strength."

Books gave Afram an escape and helped him imagine that he had his own oasis in the desert. Unfortunately, Afram's oasis was frequently disrupted.

◇

The Balcony

"CAT-ALPHA TIMES THREE, INBOUND," CORPORAL Smalls announced. "Marines ambushed with a coordinated IED attack."

He repeated the warning even louder as he rang the dreaded trauma bell incessantly.

On a Sunday, Afram thought. *Unbelievable.*

The combined casualties were by far the worst the team had seen since their arrival in Afghanistan. A total of eight Marines had been injured by IED attacks; four of them came to FOB MK, while the others went off to a higher echelon of care because of associated head injuries.

The Echo surgical team responded brilliantly to the injured Marines. More than fifty units of blood were transfused among the four victims over the twelve hours of continuous nonstop activity.

"That was awful," the usually unflappable Levine concluded after the transfer of the last patient was complete. "I don't think I've ever seen injuries that bad from so many Marines at one time."

Later that day, the commanding officer from the ambushed Marine unit personally thanked the surgeons for their work. "Without you guys," he said, "my Marines had no possible chance of surviving."

These Marines were all young men who had been systematically injured while attempting to save each other. The enemy had employed a crude but effective coordinated IED attack that capitalized on the ethos that no Marine will leave fallen comrades behind. On this occasion, all the Marines involved were harmed.

The injuries sustained by the Marines were unforgettable. The Echo Surgical Company was exhausted, their morale was low, and tension was now palpable on the team.

That night Afram escaped to a watch station on the edge of the base perimeter, a few hundred feet from the medical STP. He called this elevated perch his "balcony." During the day, he could look out on the expanse of desert valley, with a panoramic view beyond of the Hindu Kush subranges of the Himalayas. At night, Afram would gaze up at all the celestial stars of the universe.

Beautiful, Afram thought.

He noticed he had changed over the months here; he sensed he was becoming more spiritual and reconnected to the church and his Christian heart and spirit of years ago. Not only did he seek the occasional Mass services like a thirsty child, he also carried a pocket Bible with him at all times, with a copy tucked inside of his father's letter. He seldom read the book or letter, but having them close brought him comfort.

Afram prayed every day, often several times. It was a practice he had established soon after arriving at FOB MK.

He prayed for Hiral and for his unborn child. He prayed for strength to make it through his ordeal, and to return home safely to his family.

Afram spent many sunset moments in deep reflection on the balcony, and even created a mental sketch to help him remember the peaceful scene he saw. He included the majestic mountains, the hazy landscape permeated by sand-dust, the barrier walls around the medical center, and the barbed-wire fence. During this reflection, dual helicopters hovered in the air to remind Afram of his purpose, and of how casualties were delivered to FOB MK. *We're here for good,* he thought, always trying to justify for himself the work of caring for blown-up young Marines.

During this particular late-night balcony session, after such an intense day of brutal trauma cases, Afram reflected especially on the chaplain's memorable instructions about spreading the word of Christ, in the homily he had given earlier in that morning Mass with his little congregation of seven. Afram pondered those instructions. He was deeply troubled that the Marine commanding officer had expressed his thanks only to Afram and the other surgeons for saving the Marines, while Afram felt strongly that the rest of Echo Surgical Company deserved most of the credit. He felt undeserving, knowing that it was everyone's effort on the surgical team that made possible the surgeons' work.

Afram knew what he had to do.

The next morning, during the daily morning muster with the entire Echo Surgical Company present, Afram called the team close and related to them a story.

"Yesterday, the commanding officer of the Marine unit thanked Commander Chester, Lieutenant Commander Levine, and me for doing the impossible and saving his injured Marines. We thanked him—but his comments reminded me of my time on the aircraft carrier. I was on the flight deck watching flight operations. The launching and recovery of aircraft on the carrier in the middle of the ocean was like a symphony, and I was in awe.

"One of the squadron leaders was standing next to me observing his unit in action, and I said to him, 'Sir, it's amazing what your guys do!'

"And he responded, 'Doc, we wouldn't be able to do this impossible work you're watching here unless you and everyone else on this aircraft carrier did their job expertly—from the seaman recruit in the galley to the ship's navigator. All good pilots know that fact.'

"So, just like all great pilots, great surgeons also realize we couldn't make the impossible possible without all the work each of you all do. The officer meant well in thanking us three, but it's all of you guys who make us, as surgeons, look good. When a Marine is injured, it takes the corpsman in the field to place the tourniquet on perfectly. It takes the DUSTOFF crew to fly in harm's way and rescue that injured Marine while taking fire. It takes the litter bearers to run out to the flight line and successfully and safely bring the Marine into the STP. It takes the entire team in the STP/FRSS to stabilize the patient and prepare the Marine for surgery.

"It requires every Marine on the base to walk over and donate blood when needed. It takes the nurses. It takes the anesthesiologist. It takes all the corpsmen involved to finally get the Marine to the operating room table.

"When the Marine finally gets to us surgeons, our job is easy—we just have to stop the bleeding. Our job is easy because of all the work that others do. Just like the pilots who rely on all the ship's crew members to do the impossible, we as surgeons rely on all of you guys to help us fly in the OR, and to make the impossible possible, and to look good. That's the real reason why those injured Marines survived. It's because of all of you.

"Finally, I want to leave you with a quote from John F. Kennedy, as well as a challenge. Here's the quote: 'Any man who may be asked what he did to make his life worthwhile could answer with a great deal of pride, *I served in the United States Navy.*'

"And here's my challenge: I ask you to think every day about what small thing you can do in your job here at FOB MK to make the impossible possible. When we look back at our time here, each of us can proudly say with 100 percent confidence, 'Not only did I serve with my fellow shipmates and Marines, but I was responsible for making the impossible possible every day in the desert of Afghanistan. My life was worthwhile during my time at FOB MK.'"

Baby Muhammad

"WE NEED YOU, COMMANDER AFRAM!" SAID THE voice on the phone line. Afram took the middle-of-the-night call from the Role III hospital.

"We have an Afghan child with a gunshot wound to the arm and chest, and a possible heart injury," the Role III surgeon said. "We need your assistance."

A gunshot wound to the chest and a heart injury? Afram wondered what he could actually do. He knew that patients in Afghanistan do not survive gunshot wounds to the heart. All three of the *hero* patients he operated on had been shot in the heart, and none survived.

"How can I help?" Afram finally asked.

"The child is unstable, and we don't have too much time," the surgeon asserted. "You're the only heart surgeon in the region, and we need you to get here and operate on the child."

"Operate?" Afram questioned. The Role III was miles away, at least a thirty-minute helicopter ride. How did they expect him to get there in time? Hop in a cab?

"Yes, operate!" the surgeon replied. "A helo's on the way to pick you up."

Within minutes, Afram donned all his body armor, packed his weapons, and was ready. He would be flying by dreaded helicopter into the darkness of the night. Afram recalled two pilots who had died when their helo went down one night in bad weather. Afram had sat next to both pilots and spoken to them months earlier, on the chartered jumbo jet that flew them into Afghanistan when he first arrived. He had been deeply saddened by news of their deaths; it was a sobering reality of the dangers here.

Afram was filled with anxiety. He couldn't understand how anyone with an actual injury to the heart could survive long enough for him to do any good. Not knowing how he was going to help this child, he prayed.

Afram heard the familiar sounds of dual engines—a Cobra and a Huey helicopter. Both helicopters usually flew tandem, especially at night.

"Welcome aboard, sir!" said the Huey pilot as Afram boarded. "Get strapped in, sir; the ride will be a little bumpy."

Indeed, Afram knew about bumpy helicopter rides, and he wasn't looking forward to this.

At his side, Afram carried Tonya, his M4 rifle, and Sonia, his M9 pistol. Anyone leaving the boundaries of FOB MK—a.k.a. "the wire"—had to be prepared for combat even when traveling by helo.

As they flew out of the valley, Afram briefly mused how eerily similar this experience was to the many trips he took in the States to harvest organs—flying in the middle of the night to unfamiliar hospitals, and working with different and strange staff. Only this time, Afram wouldn't be bringing back the heart. This time he was flying through the night to save a heart.

After flying over the mountain ranges and arriving at the Role III hospital, Afram quickly changed into scrubs and headed to the OR, where he was greeted by the new team. "Welcome to Role III," a trauma surgeon greeted him. "The team is ready for you, and the baby is prepared and on the operating room table." Afram had a moment to glance at the child's x-ray and to look at the monitors.

"You guys have a nice setup here," Afram noted. He immediately recognized how much better this hospital was compared to the tent he and his fellow surgeons had worked in over the past several months. Afram washed his hands in a real sink and gowned up.

He approached the OR table. "Hello everyone, I'm Commander Afram. Looking forward to working with you all—let's get started." A British vascular surgeon was scrubbed in to assist Afram, and a scrub nurse was there to help them both.

Afram had never worked with this team, and he knew all eyes would be on him. He was now a seasoned combat surgeon in his familiar territory of the chest, and he knew he would need all of his skills and talents to save the life of this child—an infant boy weighing only eleven kilograms.

"Scalpel," Afram requested.

Afram made a deliberate incision on the tender skin of the child's chest. The infant had been shot through the left arm, where the bullet had fractured the child's humerus bone; bullet fragments penetrated the child's chest on the left side.

"Scissors," Afram requested. He used the scissors to divide the child's fragile sternum, and placed a small retractor to hold the chest open. The child's pericardium, the envelope surrounding the heart, was now in view.

Afram hesitated. He knew there was no turning back. The child could easily bleed out, and there was no way to put the baby on a bypass machine to support him if the heart was severely damaged and required major repair. In a child weighing so little, it would take only moments to lose all his blood and die on the operating room table.

"Blood pressure's low," announced the anesthesiologist.

"The child's pericardial sac is bulging, and there's bleeding. I'm going to open it," Afram asserted. "Get ready with blood."

Afram cut. "Quick, suction, we need suction," he ordered. "Give blood, give blood!" he yelled.

Afram cleared the blood from around the heart and quickly found the site of bleeding. He placed his finger over the small hole in the ventricle of the heart. The child's heart was the size of a plum. Gently, Afram manipulated it.

"No blood pressure!" the anesthesiologist reported.

Afram quickly released his manipulation while keeping his finger at the site of the injury. The child stabilized.

"We need you to catch up with the blood loss," Afram informed the anesthesiologist. "I've found the injury, but we'll lose more blood while I fix the hole."

"Yes sir, we're on it!" the anesthesiologist replied.

"Okay, I need a stitch, and I'll only have one shot at this."

Afram's finger was still on the hole, timing his gentle pressure with the rapid beating of the child's heart. Afram now became aware of his own elevated heart rate. The beating of the child's heart seemed in sync with his own.

He took a deep breath. "Now! Give me the stitch," he called out.

His hands moved in a blur. He quickly pulled out the small bullet fragment and stopped the bleeding on the baby's heart by placing one strategic stitch. He tied a knot in the suture with speed and grace. Then he caught his breath, realizing he had been holding it, and felt his heart rate slow down as he exhaled.

"I think we got it!" he announced with relief, smiling behind his surgical mask.

"Blood pressure improved," the anesthesiologist reported.

"Excellent. We'll need a small chest tube, and stitches for closure."

Afram and the British surgeon worked quickly to finish the procedure, then transported the child to the surgical recovery room. Before leaving the operating room, Afram—recalling his traditional quip at the end of a transplant harvest—declared to everyone, "Thank you all for your hospitality. It's been a pleasure working with everyone."

"Thank you," the nurse replied.

"Indeed, the pleasure was all ours," the anesthesiologist added.

Shortly after he arrived in the recovery room, the breathing tube was removed from the little patient, and he was breathing on his own. His vital signs were stable. Assessing the stable child, Afram felt alive again for the first time in many months. He felt his heart warmed and opened to the sight of the little child. This time, the young person under his care still had all of his extremities, and wasn't blown up.

It's much better for me to operate on the heart, he concluded.

Afram later learned that a stray bullet had hit the baby during a local Taliban conflict. Afram met the child's father, and through an interpreter, he told the father that with the operation, his injured son was now better, and his heart was fixed.

Through the interpreter, Afram asked the man, "What is the baby's name?"

"Muhammad," the father responded in Pashto. "My son's name is Muhammad." The father's eyes were sad and anxious. He looked aged, with deep vertical lines across his face. Afram imagined that each line revealed a story of some suffering in the man's life.

Afram thought about Hiral and his own son, not yet born. He wished he could be back home with them now and witness the birth.

Muhammad's father sat at the boy's bedside. He placed his hand gently on the baby's head and glanced over to Afram. The men's eyes met. The father nodded, and Afram now saw in the man's eyes gratitude and humility. Afram understood the man's nod, and the father's tender gaze upon his son delivered the universal message of a father's love for his son.

Afram turned away, holding back his tears. He thought of his unborn son, and of all the sons he'd cared for during all the months at FOB MK. *I'll get back home for my son,* he determined.

Later that evening, an intense sandstorm blew across the desert. It was still blowing as Afram boarded the helo heading back to FOB MK.

"Good evening, sir!" said the Huey pilot.

"Good evening," Afram replied. "Looks like we have some bad weather."

"We should be okay, sir," the pilot yelled over the howling wind and the noise of the Huey's engine. "We just have to make it over the mountain range, and the weather will clear up."

"Okay," Afram responded dubiously, holding tightly to the seat belt straps.

The helo took off into a swirl of sand and darkness. Afram closed his eyes tightly as the aircraft was jolted back and forth, seeming to drop and rise randomly. Finally the Huey leveled off and all was calm again. Afram opened his eyes and noticed that the mountain range was unusually close.

BOOM!

Afram heard an ear-splitting noise, then the Huey's engine went silent, and all that could be heard was the howling desert wind.

The helicopter was falling, spinning.

Afram thought only about Hiral and his son. The helicopter spun faster, and Afram felt himself falling freely. And then—there was only darkness.

PART III

To Teach

Seven Pillars of Life

AFRAM WAS IN COMPLETE DARKNESS AND silence. The only sound he heard was his own heartbeat. Thoughts swirled in his head. "What happened?" he asked himself. "Where am I?" Hoping for an answer, he found none.

He thought about Hiral, and called out, "Hiral? Hiral! Hiral!"

Afram sensed his body was weightless. Then he felt aches, cramps, and a pounding headache. Then there were chills; he was sure he had a desert fever. He felt weak, and the slightest movement brought him great pain. He slipped into a deep sleep.

Time passed, and Afram heard the sound of loud knocking, then pounding. It persisted, getting louder and louder, with intensity and purpose.

He took in a breath and choked. He coughed.

Then Afram heard a voice. "Kareem…Kareem, you are hurt."

The voice added, "Don't move now."

With that affirmation, Afram felt a pain in his right leg and reached down to touch it. He could feel nothing.

"Be still," the voice commanded.

"What— Where— Why can't I…*why can't I move?*"

"You are safe, and you'll be okay if you listen to me," the voice instructed.

"But who are you?"

"My name is Nasir, and I'm here to take care of you. I need you to be still and to rest your body. Try not to move." Then the voice added, "You were injured in the crash."

"I crashed?" Afram asked. "Yes—I remember now. I operated on baby Muhammad with the doctors. I was on my way back to FOB MK, and I heard a loud boom. But what happened to the two pilots?"

"The weather affected your helicopter, and the aircraft crashed in the mountains," Nasir said. "But you are safe with me."

"Who are you?"

"I'm the one who's taking care of you now. You're injured, and you almost died. You need to heal."

"How is Hiral? What happened to our son?"

"Try and rest now," Nasir urged.

"But what about—" Afram drifted back to sleep.

His mind was racing—he felt a pull, then a calmness overcame him. He heard the words, "No one who puts a hand to the plow and looks back is fit for service in the kingdom of God."

Afram thought deeply about those words in the context of his situation. On this night, he was wounded, he was in pain—and he heard words. *I'm scared,* Afram thought.

He tried to recite the words he heard again: "No one… plow…service…" He tried to repeat what he heard.

One word troubled Afram—the word *plow*. He was reminded of his father's haunting question: "How's life on the farm?" Afram had realized only after his father's death that he had used the farm as a metaphor for life.

"Dad?" Afram questioned. "Is that you?"

At that moment, Nasir asked Afram, "After all you've been through in your life, what does it mean to put your hand on the plow?"

"It means," Afram answered, "that I have to accept what life gives me."

"What is your plow?" Nasir asked.

"Is it my life?" Afram questioned.

"Perhaps," answered Nasir. "On a farm, the plow is both the farmer's burden and a tool." Nasir kept pressing: "Do you believe your life is your burden, your plow?"

"No, no, of course not," Afram responded. "I've been blessed with much over the years."

"Who has given you these blessings?"

Afram paused as he thought. *I have—through my own hard work.* But he then exclaimed, "God! *God* has given me my blessings in life!"

"What have been the burdens in your life?" Nasir asked.

"There are too many to count."

"Indeed," said Nasir. "Have those burdens helped you to grow?"

Afram thought about his father's death and the discovery of his father's special letter. He thought about his mother's death and her life of burdens that impelled her journey to America. Afram thought also about his own life and the events that led him to become a doctor.

"My parents shared with me wisdom that they gained through facing the burdens of their lives," he told Nasir. "For me, here in the desert, I've witnessed terrible trauma and much death."

Afram was weeping now. His torrent of tears released emotion that had been suppressed for months. Shedding a hundred tears of grief for each Marine, Afram sobbed uncontrollably.

"And what have you done here?" Nasir pressed.

"I tried to do good, to help the wounded and care for them," Afram responded through his tears.

"Have you done your work for your own glory or for the glory of the One who gave your blessings to you?"

Afram continued to weep. He knew the true answer to this question. He did good work—but not always for God. Even at times when he wanted to spread God's will with his patients, he feared he would upset those around him and make them uncomfortable. So he would pray only in silence, or sometimes not at all.

He spoke again to Nasir. "Working for God's glory is difficult, and total commitment is hard."

"Indeed," Nasir said. "And yet, isn't living a committed life to God what all Christians are called to do?"

"Yes." Afram surrendered, realizing he hadn't entirely lived up to the task.

"When you live a life committed to God," Nasir said, "and take hold of the plow and all of life's burdens, and never look back—this will upset others. But remember, no plow ever did its job without upsetting the ground and the earth beneath it."

"How can one have such total commitment?" Afram asked desperately.

"You can have that commitment by employing the one virtue you've had all these months—as you've thought about Hiral and your son, and as you gazed upon the stars in the Afghan sky from your balcony at night."

"*Faith!*" Afram cried out, with some exasperation.

"In your present place of darkness, do not despair," Nasir ordered. "You now know your path."

"I do?"

"Indeed." Nasir kept questioning: "How can you get from a place of darkness and be a good disciple of Christ?"

"With faith and commitment," Afram responded.

Nasir pressed again. "In your place of darkness and despair, how can you get back to Hiral and your son?"

"With faith and commitment," Afram answered again.

"In your place of darkness and suffering, how can you be a good son and a good father?"

"*Through faith and commitment.*" Afram spoke the words resoundingly, with joy in his voice. Enthusiasm now filled him.

"I've helped you to find the seven gifts of truth that were always in your heart," Nasir said. "Remember, you're suffering now, and wisdom only comes through suffering. Therefore the seven gifts of the heart and pillars for your life are these:

"First, *know that you are blessed.*

"Second, *believe that God gave you skills and talents to serve Him better than you serve yourself.*

"Third, *place your hand on the plow and bear your crosses in life with enthusiasm.*

"Fourth, *when you live a life committed to God, you will make a mark on this world.*

"Fifth, *when you live the committed life of God, you will upset a lot of people, but no plow has ever done its job without upsetting the earth.*

"And sixth, *in life, commitment must be total; you must not look back but only forward, and to the stars high above the heavens, while your feet remain committed to the ground.*

"And finally: *to be a good disciple of Christ, you must never give up no matter how tough the going will be.*"

◇

The Will

IT FELT AS IF MANY DAYS HAD PASSED TO AFRAM. He was unsure where he was, but he felt his strong heartbeat and knew he was still alive.

"Do you want to leave this place of darkness?" Nasir asked.

"Yes," Afram answered. "What must I do to leave?"

"Your education will be your freedom," Nasir answered.

"How will my education be my freedom?" Afram asked with frustration.

"To know the truth is not enough to free yourself from this place," Nasir admonished. "You already had within your heart the gifts of truth. To free yourself from this place, more is needed."

The truth was therapeutic for Afram, and he felt at peace. Yet he pondered what else was needed for him to be free. He didn't understand what other education he needed.

"What emotions did you see in the eyes of Muhammad's father when you told him his son was healed?" Nasir asked.

"In his eyes I saw gratitude, humility, and love," Afram responded excitedly.

"Indeed," said Nasir. "You must not only know the truth, but you must also have the proper disposition."

"What is the proper disposition?"

"You have already extolled gratitude, humility, and love when you described the emotions in the eyes of Muhammad's father. There's a direct link to gratitude and happiness. Humility is the greatest of virtues, for it prepares one to submit himself to God. Finally, when love is given as freely to others as it is to one's self, much of what is wrong in the world will be made right."

"Then how can I leave this place now?" Afram pressed.

"You've been reminded of the truth, and holding the mental faculty of gratitude, humility, and love prepares your will for freedom," Nasir said. "But there's still something needed before you can be free of this darkness and despair."

◇

Bring the Light

MORE TIME PASSED FOR AFRAM. DAYS BEGAN TO feel like weeks. His spirit and body were stronger now, and his heartbeat was still robust.

"Are you ready to leave this place of darkness and despair?" Nasir asked.

"I am," Afram said excitedly, feeling lighter now and without pain. He had received the truth and had prepared his will. But from Nasir he understood that there was still something that remained before he would be free.

"What else must I do?" Afram asked.

"The answer is in this story that I will relate," Nasir said.

"A young priest began his study at seminary in London. He did not particularly like it, because he realized it wasn't a vacation and he missed home.

"Then he went to midnight Mass, and there he heard a story. He said the story caused him to feel better about his time in London, and he pledged that he was going to use the story one day.

"Here is the story: In a town called Warrington during World War II, there was a POW camp. Like other English towns and cities, Warrington was kept in darkness at night because of possible bombing raids. This meant that all those in the town who went to Mass at night had to do so in darkness.

"One night, in the minutes leading up to midnight, people began entering the dark church, gradually filling most of the seats. Eventually, all the seats were filled except for some in the front row.

"At midnight, prison guards escorted some German POWs inside the church, and they took their seats in the front row. This was upsetting to the people, who had many loved ones in military service fighting the Germans in the war. *We've walked here through the darkness,* the people were thinking, *only to have to share this church with German prisoners!*

"Then the priest arrived, and he made an announcement: there would be no music played because the pianist was ill. This was a further disappointment, because everyone had been looking forward to hearing the music to lift their weary spirits.

"At this point, one of the German prisoners got the attention of one of the guards and communicated a message to him. The guard got the attention of the priest and whispered a message to him. The priest nodded. Then the German prisoner came up and began playing music for the Mass. The music filled the church and was described by all as magnificent. The music played by the prisoner seemed to bring light into the darkness, and lifted everyone's spirits.

"That was the story that was heard years later by the young seminary student in London. The priest who told the story went on to say that this particular night was also like the one in Warrington, as many come together to celebrate the birth of Christ. It was true all over the world, even in places like Afghanistan. All over the world on Christmas night, people paused to celebrate the birth of our Savior.

"The priest then asked the congregation, 'Why couldn't every day be like Christmas?' However, he then cautioned that this would be missing the point.

"The point to understand, he said—for all Christians in the world—was to realize how we can bring light to the world, just as the German POW did in Warrington, and just as Christ did on the night he was born. It's up to us, the priest said, because the gospel spoke of how the angel came to the smallest of men to tell them of the good news of Christ's birth. The angel didn't come to the rich and famous, or to the world leaders of the day. Instead the message was delivered to common people, to the humble and the small.

"So how can we bring the light?" Nasir continued. "We can bring the light by asking three questions of ourselves: What have I done for Christ? What am I doing for Christ? What will I do for Christ? By asking ourselves these questions, we ensure that we bring the light to the world and spread the good news of Christ."

"What else is needed?" Afram asked. "I've listened to the story. I know the truth and the gifts of my heart, and I've prepared my will with gratitude and humility and opened my heart to love." He pleaded with Nasir: "What more must I do to leave this place of darkness and despair?"

"Nothing in life will happen without action," Nasir proclaimed. "On a farm, no harvest will occur without work and action. Yes, you have the truth in your heart, and you've prepared your will with gratitude and humility, and you've opened your heart to love. Now—just as Jesus brought the light to the world—*you must take action* to make it so.

"Now you must go," Nasir concluded, "and be a good disciple of Christ, and do the work for God. And I am and will always be here to help you find your way. Act now! Act now! *Open your eyes!*"

◇

Coming Home

AFRAM OPENED HIS EYES. EVERYTHING WAS A blur. He heard the familiar beeping of monitors and attempted to look around.

His vantage point was unfamiliar. Finally he realized that he was on a hospital bed. He was a patient!

Unable to move, Afram had a tube in every orifice of his body. His right leg was immobilized and his hands were restrained. He called out but choked on the breathing tube in his neck.

The alarms blared as Afram squirmed in the bed, filled with panic.

A team of medical personnel swarmed into the room and descended upon him. He felt a cool sensation flowing into his right arm.

Just before he drifted into sleep, he read the ID badge of the nurses hovering above him: Walter Reed National Military Medical Center.

Afram was home.

PART IV

To Lead

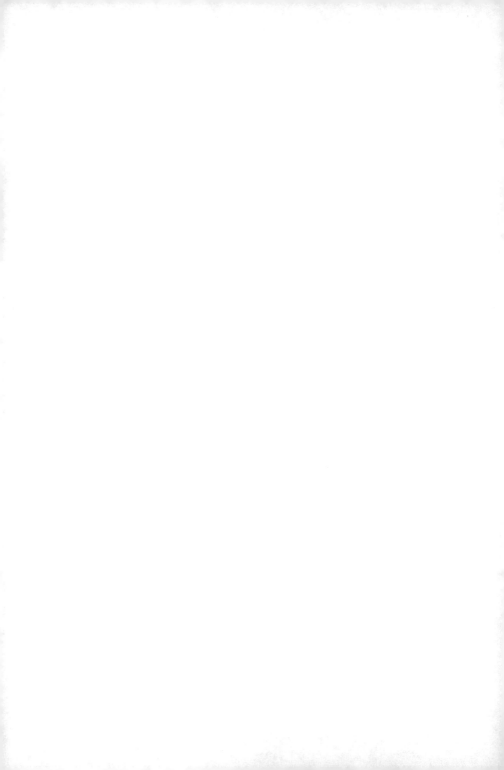

◇

Havruta

AFRAM WAS NOW MORE ALERT. HE FELT A presence of mind that he hadn't felt since the fateful night he boarded the helicopter.

"Kareem, Kareem. I'm here for you," Hiral whispered. "I'm here with you."

"Nasir?" Afram made no sound as he moved his lips.

"Kareem, my love, open your eyes—I'm with you now." Hiral squeezed his hand.

Afram slowly opened his eyes and saw her blurry silhouette. He reached out to touch her face, then touched his own.

"I see you," he whispered.

"Kareem, you crashed in the desert; your helicopter went down in the mountains. Do you remember?"

Afram was silent.

"You were lost for weeks, because you weren't found near the wreckage. The pilots didn't survive." Hiral began to cry.

Afram squeezed her hand. He tried to form his many questions for her. "But how—"

Hiral interrupted. "You were assumed killed in action, Kareem. Weeks passed, and I mourned you—but when they couldn't find your remains, I knew there was still hope, and I didn't give up on you."

Now Afram was also crying. Their tears intermixed as they wiped each other's faces and tightly squeezed each other's hands.

Hiral continued, "You were delivered to a base by a mysterious Afghan villager named Nasir. You were stripped of everything except for the small Bible in your pocket with your father's folded letter inside it. You were barely alive. This man named Nasir said he found you in the mountains on the day of the impossible eclipse, when the earth passed between the moon and the sun. He told the guards at the base that he was a friend of Muhammad's father. You slipped into a coma, and they transported you back home." Hiral didn't tell Afram that when the guards tried to detain and question Nasir, he had vanished.

"How—how long?" Afram asked in a whisper.

"You were lost to me ninety-nine days ago. Ninety-nine days! You've been in ICU for over two months. Now you're talking to me. It's a miracle!"

Afram would later learn that Hiral had kept a constant vigil at his bedside. She invited the chaplain to pray with her at Afram's side every day. They would find passages in the Bible to read aloud, and they also read the letter written by Afram's father. Some passages would make Afram move slightly or twitch, and they would repeat the passage over and over.

Hiral had studied the Bhagavad Gita as a child, and she understood helping people who struggled in the darkness was among its lessons. As a nutritionist, Hiral knew the body needed food, and she learned in her constant vigil with Kareem that he needed words for his soul and spirit that were in darkness. She believed in Karma, cause and effect, and witnessed the power the spoken words had on Kareem as he was hearing the words. Hiral prayed over Kareem, and spoke the words over and over that made him move.

Hiral never gave up hope, and Afram never met the criteria for brain death. He always demonstrated brain activity through all the testing. In addition to a significant traumatic brain injury, Afram's right leg was shattered, he had a fractured pelvis and ribs, and both arms were broken. During his hospital stay he'd been to the operating room over a dozen times to repair his injuries. Afram had a feeding tube inserted in his stomach and a tracheostomy breathing tube through a hole in his throat to help him breathe. He was a skeleton of his former self.

After several days, Afram was extensively questioned regarding the circumstances of the crash. "I don't remember anything about it," Afram told investigators, while Hiral stood patiently at his side.

"Commander Afram, surely you must remember something?" they pressed.

"I do remember speaking with Nasir," Afram said. He recalled some of his conversations with Nasir. Hiral found the story hard to believe, but fully supported Afram's assertion that someone had helped him to survive. Hiral concluded that someone had helped her husband come back home to her—and she was overwhelmingly grateful for that.

"What did Nasir look like?" the investigators inquired.

Only then did Afram realize he'd never actually seen Nasir. No one at the base could actually describe Nasir before he vanished, other than to say he was a man of the desert.

Afram's eyes had been closed the whole time he thought he was with Nasir. He recalled that he was in complete darkness throughout his entire experience with Nasir, until the moment that he opened his eyes in the hospital. Afram was frightened to realize this, and immediately uncomfortable. "Was it all a dream?" he asked himself. No, that was impossible.

Afram turned to the investigators. "I can't remember," he stated with finality and impatience.

"Commander, we need something, anything," they responded.

"You wouldn't understand," Afram told them, becoming agitated. "I never saw him, but I know he was with me—he had to be. I wouldn't have survived without him."

Noticing Afram's discomfort, Hiral excused the gentlemen, then sat next to Kareem. She tenderly caressed his forehead. Kareem reached out and gently touched Hiral's belly. Hiral smiled, "I have someone who wants to meet you!"

Hiral stepped into the hallway and waved. Hiral's mother walked in carrying her grandchild. Hiral had named their son Kwame Nasir Afram, after Kareem's father and the man who had reportedly saved her husband in the desert. "I've brought

Kwame Nasir by to see you many times, and we spoke to you and prayed for you when you were in your coma. We read your father's letter to you as well. This is the first time you've been awake long enough to see him," Hiral said.

Afram shifted in the bed, then raised his head to peek into the swaddled blanket. Hiral held Kwame Nasir close to her chest and leaned in to Afram.

Afram now saw his son up close for the first time. Mother, father, and son warmly embraced.

"Beautiful," Afram said, "Simply *beautiful*—thank you, God!" he said aloud.

◇

Life's Most Urgent Question

SEVERAL WEEKS HAD PASSED SINCE AFRAM'S awakening. Hiral, Afram, and Kwame Nasir had spent many hours reconnecting and making up for lost time.

Afram was making progress in his recovery and was gaining weight, but he was still in the hospital, on the rehabilitation floor. He was walking with assistance, increasing his strength daily.

"Commander Afram, are you making the impossible possible?" came a voice one day from the hallway outside Afram's room. The voice was familiar to Afram, but he was unable to place it exactly.

"Who is that?" he asked.

"So, sir, are you making the impossible possible?" asked the voice again—as Corporal Smalls stepped into Afram's room.

"Wow! What a surprise!" Afram said enthusiastically, happy to see a familiar face. "How are you? How's the rest of Echo Surgical Company?"

"Sir, I'm doing outstanding, I'm stationed at the Marine Corps Barracks at 8th and I, here in D.C. Almost everyone has been by to see you while you were still in your coma in ICU. Some of Echo Company are still in Afghanistan."

Afram now stood to greet Smalls.

"It's great to see you on your feet, sir," Smalls said. "Sir, I know people have asked you a lot of questions, and I won't do that—I just want to let you know we're really glad you're better, and I want to personally say thank you!"

"For what?"

"Sir, lots of people give big speeches and talk a great talk. But very few people, sir, are more than just thoughts and words. Very few people actually *do* anything."

Smalls continued, "You survived that crash and those weeks in the mountains, and made it back to your wife and son. And now you're standing—sir, you not only talked about making the impossible possible, *you did it!*"

Afram smiled, and he thought about Nasir. Afram learned that Nasir's name means "supporter" and "protector" in Arabic. Afram never saw Nasir, but Nasir had granted Afram victory and the ability to know God's truth in his heart—to prepare his will with gratitude and humility, to open his heart to love, and to take action. Nasir had conveyed wisdom to Afram, and now Afram's son, Kwame Nasir, would always remind him of that wisdom. For Afram, Nasir had illuminated life's most urgent question: *What are you doing for others and for Christ?*

Afram's brief reflective trance was broken by the voice of Smalls. "Commander Afram, sir, I know I said I wouldn't ask you this. But how *did* you do it?"

Afram knew this was his opportunity to bring the light. Afram sat down and motioned Smalls to take a seat nearby. Afram paused, took a deep breath, stared intently into the man's face, and said, "I listened to God, and I opened my eyes."

◇

Epilogue

SEVEN YEARS HAD PASSED SINCE DR. KAREEM Afram's fateful helicopter crash in the desert.

At the beginning of his extended recovery, Afram had spent several months in the military hospital in Bethesda, Maryland. During that time, Hiral and Kwame lived in a nearby hotel as Afram received rehabilitation care for his injuries. After learning how to walk again, to use his broken arms (now reconstructed with titanium rods and screws), and to maintain his memory for longer and longer conversations, Afram was finally released from the hospital.

The family traveled back to their home in Minnesota. The once familiar home environment seemed foreign to Afram, compared to the Afghan desert.

Hiral continued her important work as hospital director of surgical nutritional services. Her position was an opportunity for greater things in the future, and it paid her well.

Afram, still physically and emotionally injured from the accident and chronically traumatized from his experience, could no longer operate. The great Dr. Afram had a persistent hand tremor from his traumatic brain injury, and his eye-hand coordination was off because of his broken arms. He also experienced terrible pain from standing too long in any one spot because of his pelvic fracture that never seemed to heal just right.

"I'm not the same surgeon I was," Afram told Hiral in frustration. "I can't even remember basic steps of my operations." He attempted seeing patients in clinical consultation, but he found he didn't enjoy doctor-patient interaction as much as before since the connection didn't culminate in surgery.

Hiral and Afram visited many rehabilitation doctors and specialists all over the country, seeking help for all of Afram's problems. It was futile.

"I just want things to go back to the way they were," Afram prayed. He couldn't accept the truth that things would never again be as they were before.

Meanwhile, the family was sustained financially through Hiral's work and a generous disability policy Afram had wisely acquired early in his career.

Afram's therapist and rehabilitation doctors determined that Afram carried not only his physical injuries from the accident but also a host of mental anguish—what they called "Afram's trash."

Afram's rehabilitation physician in Minnesota was Dr. Warner, a retired naval medical officer. A seasoned veteran in his own right and a former physician to Navy SEALs, Warner regularly told Afram, "Remember Kareem, there are three options for the 'trash' you carry inside, including your self-pity and loss. You can either dump the trash on someone else, or you can get help, or you can keep the trash bottled up so that it consumes you and snuffs out any hope for future happiness."

Warner added, "I know you're seeking help—but you're keeping a lot of that trash bottled up inside, and that won't help you or anyone else in the long run. You'll need to find an outlet."

Afram listened to Warner's words—but he only listened. Nothing changed.

Hiral remained Afram's constant support. Although she was often on the receiving end of Afram's trash-dumping, she maintained a steady disposition and would remind Kareem of Proverbs 4:23: "Above all else, keep watch over your heart, for everything you do flows from it." Most importantly, on the occasions when Afram wasn't watching over his heart, *she* was. Hiral showered him with love and intimacy. They communicated constantly, and grew even closer.

Soon after they returned to Minnesota, Hiral was pregnant again. She gave birth to their second child, a daughter whom they named Kira Ivy Afram. It was only after naming her that they realized how the little girl's initials paid tribute to the many *hero* Marines killed in action. Afram had cared for many Marines in the desert who never made it back home to their families, plus many more who came back injured, their lives changed forever.

Commander Chester and Lieutenant Commander Levine both came to visit Afram and Hiral in Minnesota on several occasions, and everyone maintained a close connection, exchanging cards on holidays and birthdays. Hiral and Afram even attended Levine's wedding. His third marriage was likely the charm, and Levine proudly and happily reported the birth of his first son to his former tent mates. Chester and Afram secretly believed that they had influenced Levine's decision to finally become a family man.

Afram settled into a life of relatively insignificant existence that wore on him and his young family. He spent hours in retreat on the couch, barely helping with household chores. Only sporadically did he have the motivation to leave the house.

His son Kwame was now seven, and his daughter Kira was five.

Afram regularly thought about his experience in the desert with Nasir, the wisdom he had received, plus Nasir's challenge to do more. As Kwame and Kira played nearby, he wondered what became of baby Muhammad. Above all, he wondered what had happened to himself over all the years.

"*Life* has happened," he sadly concluded. *I was spared in the desert—but for what?* He could no longer operate and save people, and he'd spent all these years here at home wasting away on a couch while his beloved Hiral supported him emotionally.

In the midst of his thoughts, his daughter Kira ran to him to show him a paper she'd carefully folded and written on. "Daddy, this is my book," she said excitedly. "I'm writing a book to tell my friends about all the things I've learned. Do you like it?"

The question hit Afram like an energy shock. He recalled the words he used to describe his son, Kwame Nasir, so many years earlier when he was still in the hospital recovering from his injuries. "Kwame Nasir, my son, was my wisdom," Afram thought. Nasir taught him about knowing the truth and preparing the will with humility, gratitude, and love. All these years, he had thought about such things to no avail. *My circumstances haven't changed. I'm here, but I've done nothing great with my existence.*

Then he felt a sense of clarity he hadn't experienced in years. "Yet my daughter has inspired me on this day," Afram whispered to himself.

He turned to his daughter and his son and said to them, "Knowing the truth and preparing the will is not enough." They looked back at him quizzically. "*Action* is needed," he declared. "*Action* is needed! *I have to open my eyes.*"

He drew both children close in a tender embrace. "I love you both so very much. You both are my *wisdom* and *inspiration!*"

Afram quickly gathered paper and fumbled around before finally finding a pen. He began to write about what he had learned, with determination to share with everyone his message of bringing the light. Afram put the pen to paper to spread the word, and touch a million hearts.

"I will write about the truth, and extol the need to have gratitude, humility, and love to nourish the will. In doing so, I will heal, serve, teach, and lead many to the light. Denominators matter," he said with conviction, his hand cramping as he attempted to capture on paper the words flowing freely from his racing thoughts.

"I will write for the many—so that many will know the truth I hold in my heart. *Thank you, God!*"

◇

Acknowledgments

FIRST, THIS BOOK WOULD NOT EXIST WITHOUT THE service and sacrifice of all who have served our nation in uniform. I am thankful to all veterans, especially those who died and have become disabled emotionally and physically in service to our country. These individuals deserve all the care we can give.

The King James Bible is referenced. Professor J. Rufus Fears' course, *Books That Have Made History: Books That Can Change Your Life,* is credited for instruction on classical literature including the *Bhagavad Gita, On Liberty* by John Stuart Mill, and *Meditations* by Marcus Aurelius. Peter Levine's quip to Lieutenant Ryzik is adapted from Leon Trotsky's quote to Dwight Macdonald: *"Everyone has the right to be stupid, but comrade Macdonald abuses the privilege."* I am indebted to the Sailors and Marines met over the years, especially my shipmates of the Bravo Surgical Company that provided inspiration for the characters' dialogue in this work through their lively repartee and stories.

My teachers have directly and indirectly influenced this novel. Richard Lucente, Tim Penix, and Richard Robbins collectively taught me about fine literature, challenged me, and shared the power of written words. E. Thomas Moran planted early seeds of confidence and nurtured my dreams with an enduring fatherly love.

A cadre of physician mentors taught the healing art of medicine. I am especially grateful to Constance Hill, Antonio Alfonso, John Kral, Anukware Ketosugbo, Lyle Joyce, Sara Shumway, Cynthia Herrington, Rose Kelly, Kenneth Liao, John Foker, Michael Maddaus, Frederick Chen, L.D. Britt, John Thurber, Herb Ward,

R.M. "Chip" Bolman, Nelson Burton, Paul Massimiano, Alan Speir, Charles Rice, and Edward Lefrak.

At the Harvard Kennedy School, thanks to all of my professors and especially Sheila Burke, Ronald Heifitz, Linda Bilmes, Robert Blendon, and Marshall Ganz. At Johns Hopkins, I especially thank Mary Sommers, Doug Hough, and Paul Gurny.

The conceptual, editorial, and artistic work of Greg Salciccioli, Thomas Womack, Eric Weber, and Steven Dana was invaluable. Trusted sympathetic critics spent many hours with first drafts of the manuscript. Thanks to Jared Sender, Tonya Leslie, Patricia Seifert, Douglas Skopp, and Elijah Wells for their patience and support.

Surviving deployment would have been impossible if not for Michael Barker, Andy Pelczar, Jim Gennari, and Christopher Dewing. Five more different individuals could not have assembled together to share a tent and function so perfectly together to save lives in our sliver of the Afghan desert as we did. I will forever be grateful to them and to John Steely, my wingman through stateside training.

Finally, the most thanks must go to my family, and especially my wife Lisa, son Edmund, and daughter Ella for tolerating both a surgeon's and an author's schedule. Thank you all for listening at the kitchen table to endless passage recitals, for enduring many drafts and revisions, and for your patience, love, and support with tea, a special treat, and warm embrace through many long nights. You are all a blessing I am very lucky to have and thank God for every day.

Thank you to all my shipmates that care for those in harms way.
Hic Pro Bonus
Here for Good...

Hassan A. Tetteh, MD
Bethesda, Maryland

◇

About the Author

HASSAN A. TETTEH IS AN ASSISTANT PROFESSOR of surgery at the Uniformed Services University of the Health Sciences in Bethesda, Maryland. He is a thoracic surgeon and director of thoracic transplant procurement and research for Inova Health System. His clinical work includes cardiovascular disease management, treatment of heart failure, and heart and lung transplantation.

Dr. Tetteh served as ship surgeon and director of surgical services for the USS Carl Vinson (CVN 70) battle group in support of Operation Iraqi Freedom in 2005. In 2011, he deployed as a trauma surgeon to Afghanistan in support of Operation Enduring Freedom.

He is founder and principal of Tetteh Consulting Group, and is the author or subject of numerous articles in publications that include *Military Medicine*, *The Journal for Surgical Research*, *The Journal of Heart and Lung Transplantation*, *Annals of Thoracic Surgery*, *Military Officer Magazine*, and *Savoy Magazine*.

Dr. Tetteh was awarded the Alley Sheridan Award by the Thoracic Surgery Foundation for Research and Education and was named a TEDMED Front Line Scholar. He's an alumnus of the Harvard Medical School Writers' Workshop, and lives near Washington, D.C.

Dr. Tetteh is available for lectures and readings.
For information, please visit
www.doctortetteh.com
or call 800-838-7061.